624225   0208

Dr J Arumugam

MRCP (Paediatrics). Paediatric Practice Exams

1. 6, 10, 23, 33

2. 4, 5, 11, 17, 23, 28, 32

3 - 1, 4, 8, 11, 15, 16, 18, 19, 21, 22
     28, 32, 33, 34

4. 1, 2, 4, 5, 7, 8, 17, 19, 24, 25, 27
     35

5 2, 10, 13, 19, 20, 25, 26, 32, 33,
                                    35,

6 1, 5, 7, 17, 21, 22, 23, 25, 28, 32

Other Titles in the MRCP (Paediatrics) Series:

Part 1 MCQs
S Hannam, GF Fox, MJ Marsh (1996) ISBN 0 7020 1875 9

Paediatric Picture Tests
AR Craig, KG Brownlee (1997) ISBN 0 7020 2163 6

Forthcoming:

Short Cases in Paediatrics
A Glaser, J McIntyre, M Battin (1998) ISBN 0 7020 2162 8

MRCP (Paediatrics): Paediatric Practice Exams

Ian K Maconochie
MB BS MRCP
Senior Registrar
Academic Department of Paediatrics
St Mary's Hospital
Praed Street, London

Abbas Khakoo
BM BCh MRCPCH
Consultant Paediatrician
Department of Paediatrics
The Hillingdon Hospital
Uxbridge, Middlesex

Andrew P Winrow
BSc (Hons) MB BS MRCP
Consultant Paediatrician
Department of Paediatrics
Kingston Hospital
Kingston upon Thames
Surrey

WB SAUNDERS COMPANY LTD
London • Philadelphia • Toronto • Sydney • Tokyo

W. B. Saunders
Company Ltd

24–28 Oval Road
London NW1 7DX, UK

The Curtis Center
Independence Square West
Philadelphia, PA 19106–3399
USA

Harcourt Brace & Company
55 Horner Avenue
Toronto, Ontario M8Z 4X6
Canada

Harcourt Brace & Company
Australia
30–52 Smidmore Street
Marrickville, NSW 2204
Australia

Harcourt Brace & Company
Japan Inc.
Ichibancho Central Building
22–1 Ichibancho
Chiyoda-ku, Tokyo 102, Japan

A catalogue record of this book is available from the British Library

ISBN 0–7020–2381–7

This book is printed on acid-free paper

Typeset by J&L Composition Ltd, Filey, North Yorkshire

Printed in Barcelona by Grafos, S.A., Arte sobre papel

Contents

Answers

Preface

Exams are a necessary hurdle in any professional training. The MRCP looms large in the mind of the senior house officer as its achievement is vital in order to progress to specialist registrar grade and preparation for it is undertaken early in the career of the paediatrician. We hope this book of mock questions will help with this preparation and that working through it will make good use of the candidate's time, both by honing knowledge and building confidence. Two sets of written papers have been compiled by each author and comprise five case histories, ten data interpretation questions and 20 photographic slides, all of which are based on real cases. Structured answers are supplied to give the student up-to-date information and guidance on how to arrive at the correct answer. The different question styles adopted in this book reflect those that will be faced in the actual examination.

When the question requests a specific number of answers or the likeliest answer(s), these are listed at the start of the accompanying answer list. After these are listed other answers in order of decreasing merit, which will attract a corresponding decrease in the number of marks.

All three authors have been involved in teaching the MRCP exam for several years and have learnt much from successful candidates. We hope that the candidate's interest in paediatrics remains lifelong, and that he or she will look forward to learning continuously about paediatrics and get enjoyment from managing their patients for many years to come. Good luck!

IKM
AK
AW

Acknowledgements

We would like to thank Drs Shelagh Smith, Andrew Bush and Richard Kaczmarski for contributing clinical slides.

We all would also like to thank Linda Clark and Maria Khan at W.B. Saunders for being so supportive in getting this book together. Thank you both.

Abbreviations

1, 25(OH)$_2$D	1, 25-hydroxycholecalciferol
25(OH) vitamin D	25-hydroxycholecalciferol
ACTH	adrenocorticotrophic hormone
ADP	adenosine diphosphate
AIDS	acquired immunodeficiency syndrome
ALT	alanine transferase
ANA	anti-nuclear antibody
APTT	activated partial thromboplastin time
ASD	atrioseptal defect
ASOT	anti-streptolysin O titre
BCG	bacille Calmette-Guérin
BE	base excess
CH50	haemolytic complement test
CMV	cytomegalovirus
CNS	central nervous system
CPAP	continuous positive airways pressure
CRP	C-reactive protein
CSF	cerebrospinal fluid
CT	computerized tomography
DIC	disseminated intravascular coagulation
DISIDA	diisopropyliminodiacetic acid
DMSA	dimercaptosuccinic acid
DNA	deoxyribonucleic acid
dsDNA	double-stranded DNA
DTPA	diethyltriamine pentaacetic acid
EBV	Epstein–Barr virus
ECG	electrocardiogram
EEG	electroencephalogram
EMG	electromyogram
ESR	erythrocyte sedimentation rate
FBC	full blood count
FDPs	fibrin degradation products
FEF$_{25-75\%}$	forced expiratory flow 25–75% of lung volume
FEV$_1$	forced expiratory volume in one second

FiO_2	fraction of inspired oxygen
FSH	follicle stimulating hormone
FVC	forced vital capacity
G6PD	glucose-6-phosphate dehydrogenase
GnRH	gonadotrophin releasing hormone
Hb	haemoglobin
HBcAg	hepatitis B core antigen
HBeAg	hepatitis B e antigen
HBsAg	hepatitis B surface antigen
HIDA	hydroxyiminodiacetic acid
HIV	human immunodeficiency virus
HVS	high vaginal swab
Ig	immunoglobin
INR	International Normalized Ratio
IPPV	intermittent positive pressure ventilation
LDL	low density lipoprotein
LH	luteinizing hormone
LHRH	luteinizing hormone releasing hormone
MCHC	mean corpuscular haemoglobin
MCUG	micturating cystourethrogram
MCV	mean corpuscular volume
MEN	multiple endocrine neoplasia
MIBG	1, 2, 3-meta-iodo-benzyl guanidine
MRI	magnetic resonance imaging
Pa	arterial partial pressure
PCR	polymerase chain reaction
PCV	packed cell volume
PDA	patent ductus arteriosus
PEF	peak expiratory flow
PS	pulmonary stenosis
PT	prothrombin time
PTT	partial thromboplastin time
RSV	respiratory syncytial virus
SLE	systemic lupus erythematosus
T_3	triiodothyronine
T_4	thyroxine
TORCH	toxoplasmosis, other agents, rubella, cytomegalovirus, herpes simplex
TPN	total parenteral nutrition
TSH	thyroid stimulating hormone
VDRL	Venereal Disease Research Laboratories
VLDL	very low density lipoprotein
VSD	ventriculoseptal defect
WBC	white blood cell
WCC	white cell count

Introduction

The MRCP (Paediatrics) written paper is a test of clinical knowledge and has three distinct sections:

1. Four or five case histories, otherwise known as 'grey cases'.
2. Ten data interpretation questions.
3. 20 clinical pictures with matching questions.

Each one of these sections contributes one-third of the 20 marks available in the written papers; a final score of eight or less will automatically mean that the candidate will not proceed to the clinical cases and viva, which are the final components of the exam. A candidate with a score of nine will be invited to the next stage as there is the possibility that the overall score can improve sufficiently to secure a pass. For full details see 'Clinical Paediatrics for Postgraduate Examinations' by Stephenson and Wallace, published by Churchill Livingstone.

The only information given to the examiner about the candidate is his or her number.

Each section has predetermined answers and the precision of the answer is scored accordingly. Succinct terms and phrases are required, not essays on the underlying condition. Care and attention must be paid to the rubric and to the instructions given at the start of the exam.

There is no negative marking system, hence all questions must be attempted. The first answer given is the one that will be scored; therefore do not put down an extensive list of differential diagnoses.

Write legibly!

Case histories (grey cases)

The answers are to an extent dependent upon the relative prevalence of the conditions that form the differential diagnoses for the grey case. In thinking about the answer, causes that should be considered are those that are most likely, e.g. an answer of selenium deficiency as the commonest cause of cardiomyopathy in the UK may not secure full marks!

Concise answers achieve a higher score.

If you find the grey case completely bewildering – DO NOT PANIC! Take a deep breath and look at each of the clinical components of the question and for each of these compile a list of possibilities; then attempt an answer by using your full powers of deduction and best guessing.

Data interpretation

The data questions come from a limited repertoire – the candidate can expect to be asked about biochemical analysis of blood, urine, sweat and CSF. Haematological studies include full blood counts, clotting studies, platelet aggregation studies and blood films. The candidate will be expected to have a working knowledge of the normal ranges for these routine investigations.

Family trees, chromosomal studies, ECG, EEG and pH studies may also be included. There has been an increase in the number of radionuclide scans such as DTPA, DMSA and MAG 3 as well as Meckel's scans shown in this section.

Endocrine profiles may be given and their significance questioned.

Radiographs and allied investigations such as CT, MRI, ultrasound and contrast studies (e.g. MCUG) have also featured here as well as in the picture section.

Photographic material

In the picture presentations the answers are usually apparent and there may be a hint in the accompanying questions. Prepare by looking at as many slides and clinical cases as possible. Clues in the accompanying text are usually given to aid you in the direction of the answer rather than to mislead you.

And finally

To use this book effectively allocate time to sit each paper as an examination and treat each exercise as though you were sitting the real thing!

EXAM
QUESTIONS

1

2

3

4

5

6

Case History Paper

Question 1.1

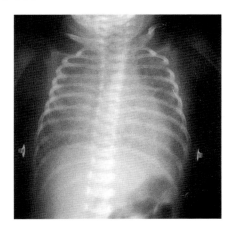

A baby boy is born at 39 weeks' gestation by emergency caesarian section due to a four-hour history of maternal pyrexia and fetal tachycardia. There has been no maternal rupture of membranes or vaginal discharge. Until this time pregnancy has proceeded uneventfully and a routine fetal anomaly scan performed at 19 weeks' gestation was normal.

The baby has Apgar scores of eight at one minute and ten at five minutes, and no resuscitation is required. No meconium is present and no respiratory distress is noted by the paediatrician attending the delivery.

The midwife becomes concerned, however, because at 12 hours of age the baby is grunting and tachypnoeic, although he remains apyrexial and feeds with no choking or coughing. The baby is therefore admitted to the neonatal unit for further assessment. Examination reveals a clinically cyanosed baby with a rectal temperature of 36.6°C, with oxygen saturation by pulse oximetry with a good trace of 82% in air. Cardiovascular examination reveals uniformly poor pulses, with a blood pressure of 40/25 mm Hg, capillary refill time of four seconds and no murmurs. Respiratory examination reveals a respiratory rate of 80 cycles per minute, intercostal recession, an expiratory grunt and fine inspiratory crackles throughout both lung fields. There is 4 cm hepatomegaly; abdominal examination is otherwise unremarkable.

The chest radiograph shown above is obtained. Analysis of right radial arterial blood gas (in air) reveals:

- pH   7.22. ↓
- Pco_2 6.8 kPa. ↑
- Po_2 4.1 kPa.
- BE   −6.8.
- O_2 saturation 81%. ↓

Blood glucose is 3.8 mmol/l.

a) What is the single most abnormal feature on the chest radiograph, and what are the blood gas abnormalities?

b) Give two possible causes of the clinical scenario given.

Question 1.2

A one-year old boy is admitted with a 24-hour history of high fever with six episodes of watery diarrhoea and approximately five episodes of vomiting during this time. His mother has been attempting to maintain his hydration with small quantities of doorstep milk on a more frequent basis, some of which has been tolerated. The mother is uncertain about his urine output as the nappies have always been stained with stools when changed.

The mother reports that the boy has previously been well other than having respiratory syncytial virus (RSV)-positive bronchiolitis at seven months of age. Since this he has had a mild cough and wheeze, which have been partially responsive to beta-agonist bronchodilator therapy delivered via a spacer and mask. He was born at term gestation with a birthweight of 3.6 kg and had no respiratory symptoms for the first seven months of life. He has a mixed diet and feeds well, and does not have any other abnormal symptoms. There are no other children in the family, and the mother, who lives alone, has not had any illness recently.

On examination the child weighs 7.1 kg and is listless, but has no focal abnormal neurological signs. Rectal temperature is 38.8°C. His peripheries are cool and capillary refill time is four seconds. Mucous membranes are dry and there is a loss of skin turgor. His pulse rate is 160 beats per minute with a blood pressure of 60/40 mm Hg. His respiratory rate is 50 cycles per minute, and there is no chest wall recession. There are occasional scattered wheezes in both lung fields, but good

1

breath sounds with no prolonged expiration and no crackles. Oxygen saturation in air is 99% on an intermittently reading pulse oximeter. Abdominal examination reveals a soft, non-distended abdomen, with no masses, no focal tenderness and active bowel sounds.

The following blood test results are obtained:

- Sodium   125 mmol/l.
- Potassium   3.2 mmol/l.
- Urea   10.9 mmol/l.
- Creatinine   98 μmol/l.
- Glucose   4.2 mmol/l.
- Hb   17.1 g/dl.
- WCC 10.3×10^9/l.
- Platelets 254×10^9/l.

a) What is the likely cause for the child's acute deterioration?

b) What is the first step in fluid management?

c) What chronic condition is most likely in this child?

Question 1.3

A two-year old boy presents with a 24-hour history of cough with noisy and fast breathing according to his mother who attends with him. The symptoms started quite suddenly in the afternoon of the previous day while the boy had been very active, playing with his toys and running about in the garden of the family home, and were not responsive to salbutamol 200 μg given four-hourly via a spacer and mask. He had previously been well, although he seemed to have a 'stuffy' congested nose, which the mother says is a regular feature. There was no witnessed choking episode and he had not initially felt hot.

In the past the boy has had mild episodes of wheezing following upper respiratory tract infections and these have been controlled with salbutamol. In between times he has no symptoms of cough or wheeze. He has otherwise been well. His father has eczema and hay fever, but there is no other family history of note.

Examination reveals an apyrexial child with a red throat and congested nasal passages with mild bilateral nasal mucosal inflammation. O_2 saturation by pulse oximetry in air is 96%, pulse rate is 120 beats per minute, and the respiratory rate is 25 cycles per minute, with reduced chest wall movement on the right side. There are reduced breath sounds at the right base and bilateral high pitched expiratory wheezes. No crackles are audible, and the rest of the examination is normal.

An initial chest radiograph shows mild hyperinflation of the left side, but no other focal abnormalities. After 24 hours of nebulized beta-agonist therapy, the boy continues to have a persistent cough, and he develops a pyrexia of 38°C. Chest examination remains as before, although there are fewer rhonchi, and a few crackles are audible at the right base posteriorly. O_2 saturation is 94% in air. A repeat chest radiograph shows an area of consolidation with volume loss in the right lower lobe and he is started on intravenous antibiotics.

a) What is the diagnosis in this boy?

b) What urgent intervention must now be performed?

Question 1.4

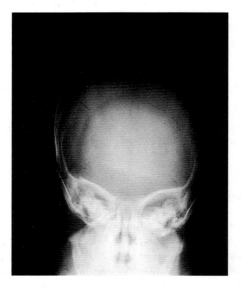

A two-month-old baby girl is brought to the accident and emergency department by her parents with a story of having rolled off a bed two days before, with a bruise appearing over the right side of the head a few hours later. She has been increasingly irritable and has been feeding poorly and vomiting since.

Further questioning of the parents reveals two previous accident and emergency department attendances since the baby's birth for excessive crying and difficult feeding, as well as several attendances to the general practitioner for the same problem. The parents have been given a diagnosis of 'colic'. There have been no other symptoms, she is physically thriving and she has recently had her first vaccination. The birth history was normal, and mother and baby were discharged home when she was 24 hours of age, bottle feeding having been well established.

The parents have been together for five years, and had a previous child who died of apnoea two years before at 15 months of age. They are extremely concerned that this child may have the same condition.

Examination reveals an irritable child with a full anterior fontanelle and a bruise over the right temporo-parietal region, but no focal neurology. Pupils are mid-point in size and equal and both react to light. Blood pressure is 90/64 mm Hg, and pulse is 104 beats per minute with normal cardiac auscultation. The child has normal growth parameters with no other obvious skin or bone lesion on full examination except a subcutaneous lump at the site of the recent vaccination. Respiratory, abdominal and ear, nose and throat examinations are normal.

A skull radiograph requested by the casualty officer is shown opposite.

a) Name two abnormalities shown on this radiograph.

b) What further radiological imaging is indicated in the light of the clinical story and this skull radiograph?

c) What three further steps are essential in the further assessment of this baby?

d) What is the most likely diagnosis?

Question 1.5

A term female infant is delivered vaginally weighing 3.4 kg. Her heart rate is over 100 beats per minute at one minute of age, and she cries at birth, with regular respirations being established immediately. Her Apgar score is eight at one minute. This is her mother's third pregnancy, and the pregnancy has been followed up solely by her general practitioner, who has had no concerns. The labour has been uneventful with no evidence of fetal distress, no risk factors for maternal infection, and no meconium staining of the liquor.

Within a few minutes the baby girl has evidence of respiratory distress, with chest wall recession and cyanosis. Despite intermittent positive pressure ventilation (IPPV) via a bag and mask device with a good facial seal the baby's condition does not improve and chest wall movement is poor.

a) What are the next two steps in resuscitation?

Continuing **IPPV** chest auscultation reveals reduced breath sounds, particularly on the left side, and heart sounds are best heard on the right side.

b) Name two differential diagnoses that must now be considered.

c) Name one clinical clue and one simple bedside test that may help distinguish between these conditions.

Data Interpretation Paper

Question 1.6

An eight-year-old girl presents with a short history of leg cramps. Results of investigations are as follows:

- Hb   13.4 g/dl.
- WCC 13.8×10^9/l.
- Platelets 354×10^9/l.
- Sodium   134 mmol/l.
- Potassium   3.9 mmol/l.
- Urea   5.2 mmol/l.
- Serum osmolality   298 mOsm/kg.

a) What further investigation would you request?

b) What is the diagnosis?

Question 1.7

An 11-year-old child of average build is seen in the chest clinic with the following spirometry:

	Predicted	Measured	%
FVC (1)	2.74	2.69	98
FEV_1 (1)	2.51	1.82	72
FEV_1/FVC (%)	91	68	−23
PEF (1/min)	350	252	71
$FEF_{25-75\%}$ (1/s)	3.00	1.37	45

a) What pattern of lung disease is suggested by the spirometry?

b) What further spirometry should be performed to help achieve a diagnosis?

Question 1.8

The following cardiac catheter data are obtained from a four-month-old child with breathlessness, failure to gain weight and a heart murmur:

	Oxygen saturation (%)	Pressure (mm Hg)
Superior vena cava	70	
Inferior vena cava	75	
Right atrium	73	mean 3
Right ventricle	85↑	45/5–8↑
Main pulmonary artery	85 ↑	45/25 mean 37↑
Pulmonary vein	98	
Left atrium	98	mean 6
Left ventricle	98	120/80–10 ↑
Ascending aorta	98	75/50 mean 60
Descending aorta	98	76/49 mean 60

a) What two cardiac lesions are suggested by these cardiac catheter data?

Question 1.9

A newborn baby is cyanosed from birth. The following investigation results are obtained at four hours of age:

Good bubble-free arterial blood gas (left radial artery) in headbox oxygen with FiO_2 0.8.

- pH   7.38.
- $Paco_2$ 4.2 kPa.
- Pao_2 48.0 kPa.
- Oxygen saturation 99.5%.

Pulse oximetry (good trace) left hand.

- O_2 saturation   70%.
- Hb   14 g/dl.

a) What is the most likely diagnosis?

b) What simple bedside test may aid diagnosis?

c) Name two commonly used therapeutic agents in this condition.

Question 1.10

A seven-year old boy is involved in a road traffic accident. On arrival in the accident and emergency department he is unconscious and pulseless and has the ECG shown below.

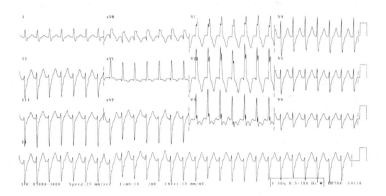

a) What is the diagnosis?

b) Name the three urgent steps in initial resuscitation.

c) Name three possible causes in this case.

Question 1.11

The following blood test results are obtained as part of a failure to thrive screen in a one-year old Greek boy:

- Hb   11.2 g/dl.
- MCV   70 fl.
- Mean corpuscular Hb   25 pg.
- MCHC   29 g/dl.
- Hb electrophoresis   Normal.
- HbA_2 2% (normal).
- Serum ferritin   30 ng/ml (normal).

a) What two abnormalities are present?

b) What is the likely diagnosis?

c) What is the clinical significance of this condition?

Question 1.12

A 14-year-old girl with cystic fibrosis has a two-week history of increased breathlessness with significant wheezing and clear sputum production. The following results are obtained:

- Total IgE 1200 IU/ml (previously 150 IU/ml on annual assessment blood tests three months previously).
- Hb   11.8 g/dl.
- WCC $11.4 \times 10^9/l$ (60% neutrophils, 30% lymphocytes, 10% eosinophils).
- Platelets $234 \times 10^9/l$.
- Sputum culture   Negative.

a) What is the likely diagnosis?

b) What may a chest radiograph show?

c) What is the treatment?

Question 1.13

A two-year-old Caucasian boy is investigated for failure to thrive and persistent diarrhoea. Among the investigation results are the following:

- CD4+ count $0.3 \times 10^9/l$.
- CD8+ count $1.2 \times 10^9/l$.
- Total lymphocyte count $3.2 \times 10^9/l$.
- IgA   2.3 g/l
- IgG   16.0 g/l
- IgM   2.4 g/l

a) What do these results show?

b) What further investigation must be performed?

Question 1.14

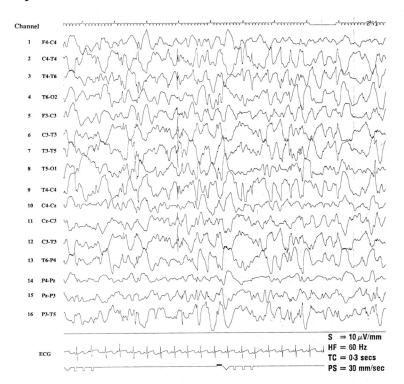

The EEG shown above was taken from a nine-month-old child with Down syndrome.

a) What abnormality is shown?

b) What seizure type is associated with this EEG?

Question 1.15

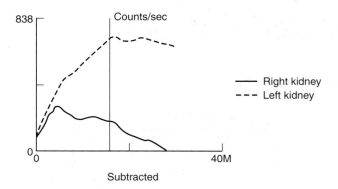

The DTPA (diethyltriamine pentaacetic acid) renogram shown above is from a five-year-old boy with recurrent left-sided abdominal pain. Frusemide was given 16 minutes into the study.

a) What does the renogram show?

b) Name one renal tract abnormality that may present in this way.

Photographic Material Paper

Question 1.16

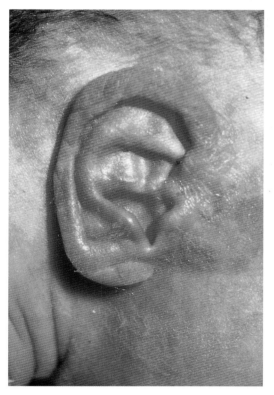

a) What is the abnormality shown, and with what syndrome is it associated?

b) What is the most serious complication seen in the neonatal period?

Question 1.17

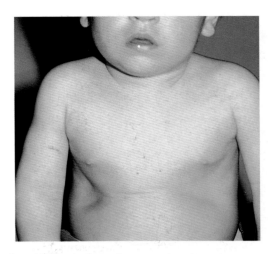

a) What abnormality is shown?

b) In what condition is this most commonly seen?

Question 1.18

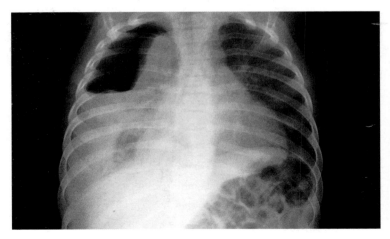

a) Name three abnormalities seen on this chest radiograph.

b) What is the likeliest aetiology?

Question 1.19

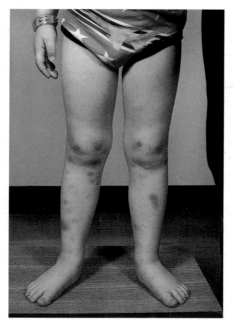

This rash appeared four days after an upper respiratory tract infection in an otherwise well child, and was also present on the buttocks.

a) What is the likeliest diagnosis?

b) Name two laboratory investigations that will guide treatment and prognosis.

Question 1.20

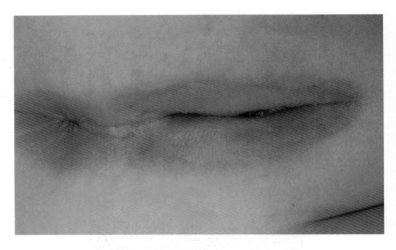

This perineal rash was seen in a six-year-old girl seen in outpatients with a three-month history of abdominal pain.

a) Name two possible diagnoses.

Question 1.21

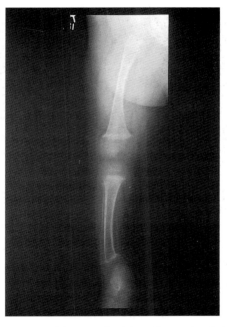

a) Name four abnormalities seen in this radiograph of the leg bones of an eight-month-old baby boy seen with a fracture following an accidental fall.

b) What is the diagnosis?

c) Name three other clinical features likely to be present on examination of this child.

Question 1.22

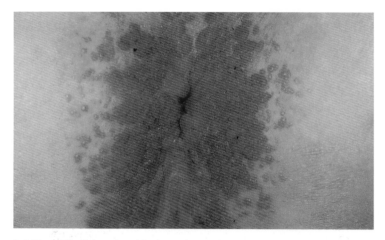

a) What are the perineal lesions shown in this two-year-old boy?

b) What causative factor must be excluded?

Question 1.23

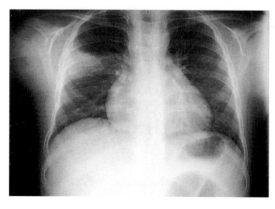

A three-year-old boy with a small ventricular septal defect has a fever, cough and chest pain. His chest radiograph is shown above.

a) What complication has occurred?

b) How can the diagnosis be most easily confirmed, and what will it show?

Question 1.24

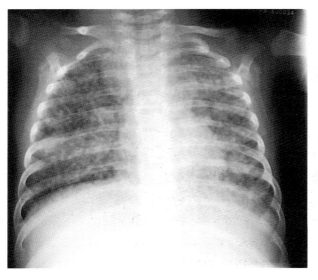

This four-month-old boy of Pakistani origin had a two-week history of fever and irritability and a three-day history of breathlessness. Examination reveals a tense anterior fontanelle and bilateral lung crackles. His chest radiograph is shown above.

a) What is shown on this chest radiograph?

b) Name two tests that may help confirm the diagnosis.

Question 1.25

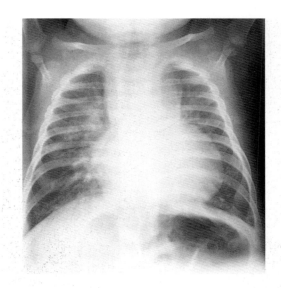

This six-month-old child became breathless and pale and developed respiratory difficulty ten days after a coryzal illness associated with diarrhoea and a low-grade fever.

a) Name two abnormalities shown on this chest radiograph.

b) What is the likely diagnosis?

Question 1.26

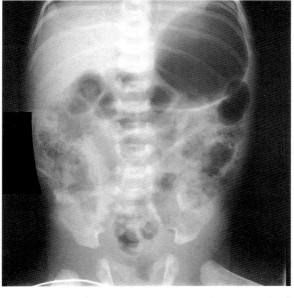

This preterm baby became unwell with abdominal distension and bile-stained vomiting.

a) What is the major abnormality seen on this plain abdominal radiograph?

b) What is the diagnosis?

Question 1.27

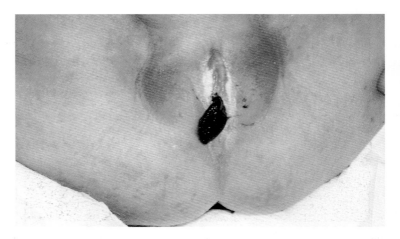

a) Name two abnormalities shown above.

Question 1.28

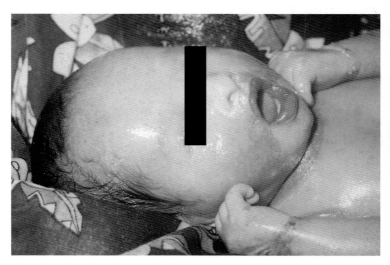

a) What is this condition?

b) Name two important complications that may occur in the neonatal period.

Question 1.29

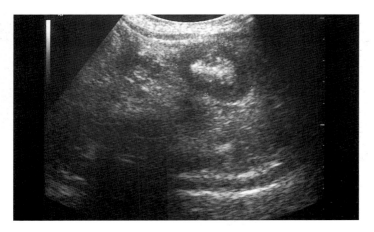

This nine-month-old baby boy presented with an 18-hour history of drawing up his legs and vomiting.

a) What does this abdominal ultrasound show?

Question 1.30

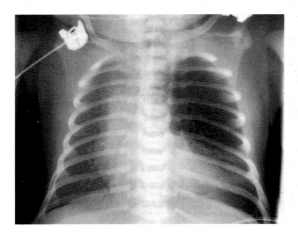

This newborn baby developed respiratory distress with tachypnoea at two days of age.

a) What is the most likely diagnosis?

Question 1.31

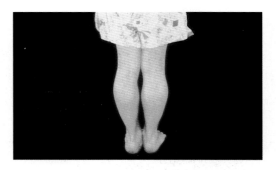

This four-year-old boy presented with difficulty walking upstairs.

a) What physical sign is shown?

b) What is the likely diagnosis?

c) Name three tests that will help confirm the diagnosis.

Question 1.32

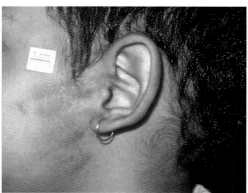

This lesion was noticed incidentally by a schoolteacher at this child's school.

a) Give a possible explanation for the appearance.

Question 1.33

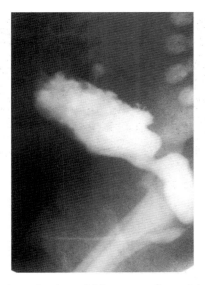

a) What is this investigation which was performed in a three-day-old baby boy?

b) Name three abnormalities and the diagnosis.

Question 1.34

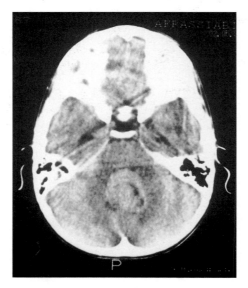

a) Name two abnormalities shown on this cranial CT scan.

Question 1.35

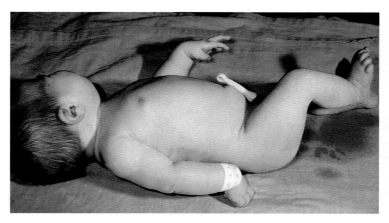

a) What is wrong with this newborn infant?

b) What maternal medical condition predisposes to this abnormality?

EXAM QUESTIONS

1

2

3

4

5

6

Case History Paper

Question 2.1

A four-year-old girl, usually resident in the UK, presents with a four-month history of limping and difficulty in weightbearing on the right leg, which began one month into a three-month summer holiday visiting relatives abroad. She had otherwise appeared well with no obvious fever at that time. There had been no history of trauma at around the time at which the symptoms began, and no other musculoskeletal symptoms subsequently. She was started on ibuprofen with good symptomatic relief. Her stay abroad was complicated only by an episode of diarrhoea and vomiting in the last month of her holiday. This lasted for three days with quick and complete resolution of fever and gastrointestinal symptoms. Since returning to the UK two months ago, she has developed swelling of the right wrist resulting in reduced function.

This girl has otherwise been healthy, up-to-date with all routine vaccinations and with no preceding joint symptoms. The whole family had consulted a local travel clinic before the holiday and all recommended precautions had been taken. Her grandmother had scleroderma, and her mother was receiving regular physiotherapy for back pain. While abroad one of the elderly relatives she was staying with began treatment for suspected pulmonary tuberculosis.

Examination shows a well-looking girl with an axillary temperature of 37.2°C. Chest, cardiovascular and abdominal examinations are all normal. Blood pressure is 95/65 mm Hg. There are no skin rashes and musculoskeletal examination is normal except for swelling and limited movement of the right knee and right wrist, with mild warmth of both joints, but no overlying erythema.

The results of investigations are as follows:

- Hb   9.8 g/dl.
- WCC 14.1×10^9/l (60% neutrophils, 39% lymphocytes).
- Platelets 420×10^9/l.
- Blood film   Normal.
- CRP   20 mg/l.
- ESR   28 mm/h.

- Heaf test negative.
- Chest radiograph normal.
- Right wrist and knee radiographs – soft tissue swelling, otherwise normal.
- Urine microscopy and culture normal.
- Early morning urine dipstick 2+ protein.

a) What is the likeliest cause of the musculoskeletal problems?

b) What investigation would help confirm the diagnosis and what further screening must be performed?

c) Give two causes for the urine findings.

Question 2.2

A mother with gestational diabetes mellitus has a full-term normal vertex delivery and her baby weighs 4.2 kg. Control of the maternal diabetes mellitus on insulin has been variable during the pregnancy, the last maternal HbA_{1C} being 7.0, and pregnancy has been otherwise uncomplicated. During labour there have been no particular concerns about fetal well-being, no risk factors for infection and no meconium-stained liquor. The head is delivered without difficulty, but there is some difficulty in delivering the rest of the body according to the midwife performing the delivery.

The baby cries immediately after birth, and requires no resuscitation. Heart rate is over100 beats per minute by one minute of age, and by this time the baby is pink with good tone. Respiratory rate at one minute is 70 cycles per minute. The Apgar score is nine at one minute. However, soon after birth the whole of the left arm is noted to have reduced movements and is held in an adducted position.

a) Name two possible causes of the reduced movements of the left arm.

After 20 minutes of age, the baby continues to have a respiratory rate of 70 cycles per minute and O_2 saturation in air as determined by pulse oximetry is 90%. Chest examination reveals reduced breath sounds over the left hemithorax, most marked at the left lung base posteriorly. There are no added sounds, and clinically there is no mediastinal shift. The cardiovascular, abdominal and remaining neurological examinations are all normal. A chest radiograph is requested.

b) What abnormality may the chest radiograph show in this case?

c) What further radiological imaging is needed to confirm the respiratory diagnosis?

Question 2.3

A 14-year-old West African boy who is usually resident in London returned two days ago from a three-week holiday in West Africa. He did not take his antimalarials while there due to the unpleasant taste of the medication, and no other specific travel precautions were taken other than the compulsory yellow fever vaccination. Five days before returning to England, he developed a fever and headache, a clinical diagnosis of malaria was made and a course of chloroquine prescribed. Despite this he has continued to remain unwell with persistent fever, frontal headache, cough, vomiting and abdominal pain. He last passed a stool three days ago and he has no other gastrointestinal symptoms. A seven-year-old sibling developed a diarrhoeal illness while accompanying him, but this settled with oral rehydration within 48 hours.

Usually he is a well boy, though he has mild asthma controlled on a low dose of inhaled steroids and mild eczema managed with emollients only. He was born at 36 weeks' gestation and was on the special care baby unit for the first seven days of life with feeding difficulties requiring nasogastric feeds and phototherapy for jaundice from day 2 to day 6. There is no relevant family history of note.

On examination, the boy is pyrexial at 39.8°C, there are no enlarged lymph nodes, and ear, nose and throat examinations are normal. The sclerae are yellow tinged, the mucous membranes are dry, there are no visible rashes or bite marks, and capillary refill is one second. The pulses are of good volume at a rate of 74 beats per minute. Blood pressure is 108/70 mm Hg and heart sounds are normal with no murmurs. Chest examination reveals some scattered crackles, but no other abnormalities. Abdominal examination reveals a tender 3 cm enlarged spleen. Although a little lethargic, there is no impairment of conscious level and no meningism or focal neurological signs.

The results of investigations are as follows:

- Hb — 6.8 g/dl.
- WCC — 5.6×10^9/l (neutrophils 20%, lymphocytes 79%, monocytes 0.5%).
- Platelets — 167×10^9/l.
- Blood smear (thick and thin) — No malarial parasites seen.
- Prothrombin time — 14 s (control 13 s).
- Alanine aminotransferase — 20 IU/l.
- Alkaline phosphatase — 130 IU/l.
- Total bilirubin — 56 μmol/l.
- Conjugated bilirubin — 2 μmol/l.

- Urinalysis   4+ urobilinogen, 2+ protein.
- Urine microscopy and culture   Normal.
- Chest radiograph   Mild bilateral interstitial
                                            shadowing.

a) What is the most likely cause of the febrile illness?

b) What haematological complication has occurred?

c) What factor in this child may have predisposed him to this complication?

Question 2.4

A mother vaginally delivers a term + 6 days baby boy, with a birthweight of 3.2 kg. At birth the baby is pale and limp with no spontaneous
movements. There is no spontaneous respiratory effort and intermittent
positive pressure ventilation is commenced via bag and mask. Heart
rate is 60 beats per minute at birth.

This is the mother's first pregnancy and it has been uncomplicated until
labour. There have been no indicators of maternal infection, no ante-
or intra-partum haemorrhage, and the membranes ruptured 18 hours
before delivery. At this time there was meconium staining of the liquor,
but cardiotocographic monitoring was unremarkable. The second stage
of labour lasted 25 minutes. Umbilical artery cord pH was 7.1.

At three minutes of age the baby is intubated and IPPV is commenced
with oxygen. Good bilateral breath sounds and expansion are present.
No meconium is seen at the level of the vocal cords during intubation.
Five minutes after the birth irregular respirations are established and
the heart rate is approximately 120 beats per minute. By ten minutes of
age the baby has more regular respirations with a respiratory rate of 70
cycles per minute; chest examination is otherwise normal and the baby
is extubated. Rectal temperature is 36.5°C. Tone is still poor, but the lips
are now pink. Analysis of arterial blood gas in air at this time shows the
following:

- pH   7.20.
- P_{CO_2} 3.2 kPa.
- P_{O_2} 9.8 kPa.
- Bicarbonate   12.2 mmol/l.
- BE   -15.8 mmol/l.

a) What does the arterial blood gas show?

b) What two further important pieces of information about the baby's
condition are urgently needed?

Following stabilization on the neonatal unit, at two hours of age the baby becomes extremely irritable, with increased tone in all four limbs. Intravenous 10% dextrose is commenced at 60 ml/kg/day. At 12 hours of age, intermittent rhythmic jerking of all four limbs with occasional 'cycling' movements of the legs is noted, during which the baby becomes cyanosed with irregular respirations. At this time the anterior fontanelle is noted to be full and non-pulsatile. A cranial CT scan is performed at this time and is shown below.

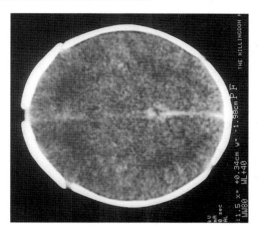

c) What is the single most important feature shown on the cranial CT scan?

d) Name two important urgent biochemical assessments that must now be made.

e) What is the likely primary diagnosis in the baby?

Question 2.5

A five-year-old boy presents acutely to the accident and emergency department with a five-day history of fever, diffuse rash, sore throat and abdominal pain. He has had some vomiting and loose non-bloody stools over the same period of time. The general practitioner was consulted on day 2 and on finding a red throat had started treatment with penicillin V. Despite this the fever has continued, and the boy's eyes have also become very red. At the time of presentation the boy complains of increasing lethargy, general muscular aches and pains, and poor appetite.

There has been no recent travel abroad and no one else in the family has been unwell recently. The boy is up-to-date with all his vaccinations for his age, and has no relevant past medical history of note. He has in the past taken amoxycillin for an episode of tonsillitis without any adverse reaction.

On examination, he is pyrexial with a temperature of 39.4°C. He has a diffuse macular rash, which is most marked over the trunk, and no petechiae. He has a bilateral conjunctival injection and his sclerae are tinged yellow. He has a redness of his lips and oropharynx, but his tonsils are not significantly inflamed, and there is no exudate or pus. A few cervical lymph nodes are palpable, the largest being 1.5 cm in diameter, and no other lymphadenopathy. His peripheries are cool, capillary refill time is four seconds and his pulse is 160 beats per minute; all pulses are reduced in volume. Blood pressure is 70/46 mm Hg. Heart sounds are normal and there is a soft ejection systolic murmur best heard at the left sternal edge with no radiation, no palpable thrill and no accompanying clicks. Respiratory rate is 30 cycles per minute and chest examination is normal. Abdominal examination reveals mild diffuse tenderness, but no guarding, and 3 cm of hepatomegaly, but no splenomegaly. He has mild lethargy, no meningism, and no focal neurological signs.

The results of investigations performed are as follows:

- Throat swab   No growth.
- Urine microscopy and culture   > 100 white cells/ml.
                                         No growth
- Urinalysis   2+ proteinuria.
- Stool cultures   Negative.
- Blood cultures   Negative.
- Hb   12.1 g/dl.
- WCC 19.6×10^9/l (85% neutrophils, 14% lymphocytes).
- Platelets 98×10^9/l.
- Blood film   Normal.
- PT   17 s (control 14 s).
- ESR   56 mm/h.
- CRP   72 mg/l.
- Sodium   138 mmol/l.
- Potassium   4.6 mmol/l.
- Urea   6.0 mmol/l.
- Creatinine   36 µmol/l.
- Total bilirubin   45 µmol/l.
- Alanine aminotransferase   55 IU/l.
- Alkaline phosphatase   145 IU/l.

a) Name the two conditions that are most likely to be responsible for the child's illness.

b) Name three further investigations that can help in differentiating between the two conditions.

2

Data Interpretation Paper

Question 2.6

A 14-year-old boy with a repaired lumbosacral myelomeningocoele complains of a three-month history of anorexia and vomiting. The following blood biochemistry is obtained:

- Sodium   138 mmol/l.
- Potassium   5.5 mmol/l.
- Urea   46.4 mmol/l.
- Creatinine   275 micromol/l.
- Glucose   4.4 mmol/l.
- Calcium   2.0 mmol/l.
- Phosphate   2.3 mmol/l.
- Albumin   44 g/l.
- Alkaline phosphatase   1100 IU/l.

Urine culture reveals over 10^5 coliforms per ml.

a) What two abnormal physiological processes are indicated by the history and electrolytes?

b) What is the aetiology in this case?

c) Give the two most important steps in the immediate management.

Question 2.7

A five-month-old boy with poor appetite and poor growth has the following blood biochemistry:

- Sodium   132 mmol/l.
- Potassium   2.9 mmol/l.
- Urea   3.6 mmol/l.
- Creatinine   38 µmol/l.
- Chloride   114 mmol/l.
- Bicarbonate   12 mmol/l.
- Arterial pH   7.15.
- Urine pH   5.0.

a) What diagnosis is suggested by these results?

b) Name two other urinary biochemical abnormalities that should be sought.

Question 2.8

A three-month-old baby boy is admitted with hypernatraemic dehydration. Following recovery a six-hour fast is planned. However, this is stopped at four hours and the following results are obtained.

	Duration of fast (h)	
	0	4
Body weight (kg)	3.51	3.34
Blood biochemistry (mmol/l)		
Sodium	138	145
Potassium	4.0	4.5
Glucose	4.0	3.0
Urea	2.0	3.0
Urine osmolality (mOsm/kg)	120	140

a) What is the diagnosis?

b) What is the next investigation that should be performed?

Question 2.9

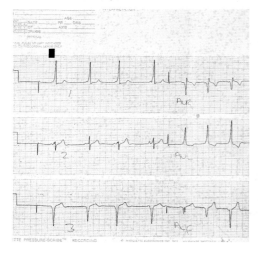

This ECG was taken from a nine-month-old child following recovery after an episode of cardiac failure.

a) Name three abnormalities.

b) What is this constellation of abnormalities commonly called?

Question 2.10

A four-day-old full-term baby born by elective caesarian section who is breastfed presents with an episode of rectal bleeding, but is otherwise well. The following results are obtained:

- Hb   13.4 g/dl.
- WCC 9.6×10^9/l.
- Platelets 254×10^9/l.
- PT   13.4 s (control 14.1 s).
- APTT   32 s (control 34 s).
- Apt test on baby's stool   Positive.

a) What is the cause of the baby's rectal bleeding?

Question 2.11

A four-day-old baby boy is noted to have poor feeding and lethargy. Examination does not reveal any specific abnormalities. The results of the investigations performed are as follows:

- Septic screen   Negative.
- Plasma sodium   140 mmol/l.
- Plasma potassium   3.9 mmol/l.
- Plasma urea   0.8 mmol/l.
- Plasma creatinine   48 μmol/l.
- Blood glucose   2.6 mmol/l.
- Plasma ammonia   600 μmol/l.

The analysis of arterial blood gas in air reveals:

- pH   7.44.
- pCO_2 3.9 kPa
- pO_2 15.5 kPa.
- Bicarbonate   20.8 mmol/l.
- BE -2.

a) What metabolic pathway is most probably deranged in this baby?

b) Name two further investigations that will help delineate the enzyme defect further.

Question 2.12

This ECG is taken from a three-day-old baby.

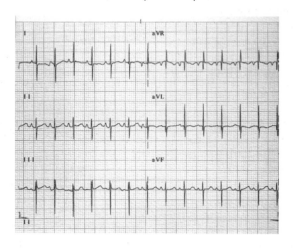

a) What is the single major abnormality shown?

b) Name two cardiac abnormalities that may present in this way.

Question 2.13

A four-month-old baby boy presents with a short history of vomiting, lethargy and being floppy. He has just commenced on a weaning diet, having been exclusively breastfed until then. The results of investigations performed are as follows:

- Septic screen   Negative.
- PT   98 s (control 13 s).
- Bilirubin   48 μmol/l.
- Alanine aminotransferase   120 IU/l.
- Alkaline phophatase   220 IU/l.
- Albumin   20 g/l.
- Blood glucose   1.6 mmol/l.

a) What is the likely diagnosis?

b) How is the definitive diagnosis made?

c) What is the long-term treatment?

Question 2.14

A 28-week-gestation neonate, now four days of age, is being ventilated for hyaline membrane disease, with good gas exchange and no evidence of circulatory failure. For ease of access, he has been nursed under an overhead radiant heater since birth, and since day 3 has been receiving phototherapy. He is currently receiving total fluids of 150 ml/kg/day, this having been increased in increments of 30 ml/kg/day from 60 ml/kg/day on day 1. The fluid has had no added sodium since day 1. He has the following biochemistry.

Day	1	2	3	4
Plasma				
Sodium (mmol/l)	135	145	152	155
Potassium (mmol/l)	4.2	3.8	4.0	5.2
Urea (mmol/l)	3.5	3.6	4.6	5.8
Creatinine (mmol/l)	65	68	88	94
Glucose (mmol/l)	3.5	6.2	10.0	12.5
Albumin (g/l)	25	28	30	30
Urine				
Glycosuria (%)	0	1.0	1.5	1.5

a) Give two reasons for the abnormal plasma biochemistry.

b) Give three principles for correcting the abnormalities.

Question 2.15

A four-month-old baby with an acute rotavirus gastroenteritis four weeks previously presents with persistence of loose stools. Feeding has been exclusively with a cow's milk-based infant formula. The results of investigations are as follows:

- Stool pH   4.5.
- Stool reducing substances (Clinitest)   1.5%.
- Stool cultures (bacteriology and virology) Negative.

a) What is the most likely diagnosis?

b) What is the appropriate therapy?

Photographic Material Paper

Question 2.16

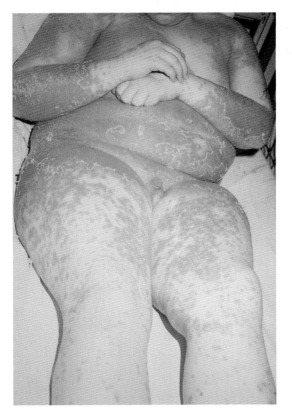

a) What has occurred in this 14-year-old boy with mild atopic eczema?

b) Name three lines of treatment.

Question 2.17

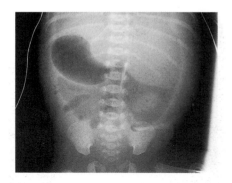

a) Name two abdominal abnormalities in this abdominal radiograph of a four-day-old baby with a two-day history of abdominal distension.

b) What underlying condition most commonly results in this appearance?

Question 2.18

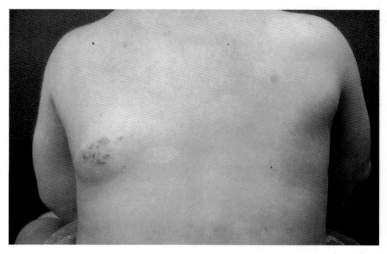

a) What is the diagnosis?

b) What is the eventual outcome of this lesion?

Question 2.19

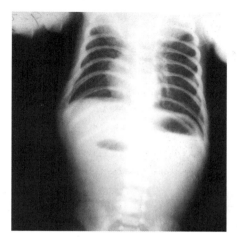

2

a) What is the diagnosis?

b) With what syndrome is it associated?

Question 2.20

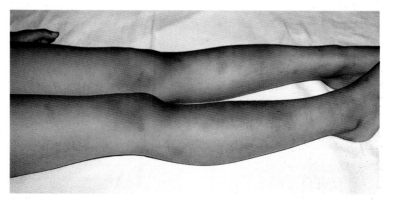

a) What is the name of these painful lesions?

b) Name four conditions with which they are associated.

Question 2.21

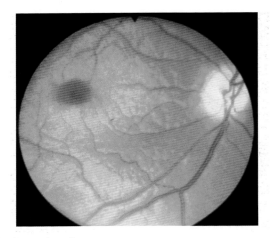

a) What is shown here?

b) Name two conditions with which this finding is associated.

Question 2.22

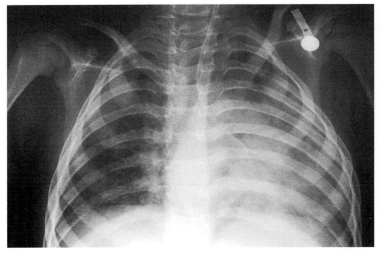

a) What is the diagnosis in this child with cerebral palsy and pseudobulbar palsy who presents with respiratory distress?

Question 2.23

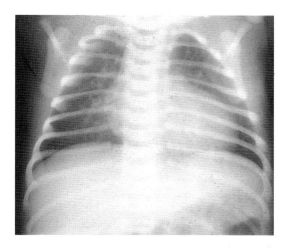

2

This neonate presented with cyanosis at 12 hours of age, with no abnormal respiratory findings and no cardiovascular abnormalities other than a single second heart sound.

a) Name three abnormalities seen on this chest radiograph, and the likely diagnosis.

b) What is the reason for the single second heart sound?

Question 2.24

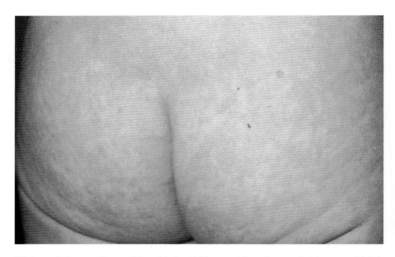

This rash is seen in an 18-month-old boy with a six-week history of high fever, hepatosplenomegaly, and difficulty in walking.

a) What is the diagnosis?

Question 2.25

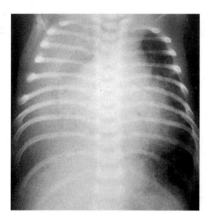

a) What complication has occurred in this two-week-old baby with cyanotic congenital heart disease requiring a right modified Blalock-Taussig shunt?

Question 2.26

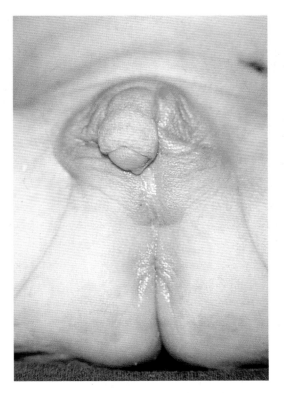

2

These external genitalia are noted on a routine 24-hour neonatal check.

a) What single important clinical sign must be elicited?

b) What is the most common and serious condition to exclude when this appearance is seen and why?

Question 2.27

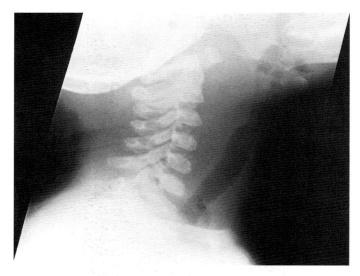

This 14-month-old presented with high fever, difficulty in swallowing and inspiratory stridor.

a) What is shown on this lateral neck radiograph?

b) What is the likely diagnosis?

Question 2.28

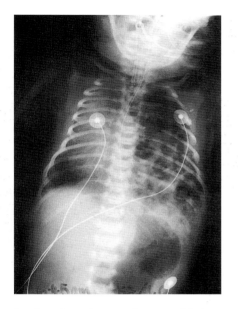

2

This newborn developed respiratory distress at birth.

a) What is the most likely diagnosis with this sort of appearance?

b) In this case what further investigation may be useful?

Question 2.29

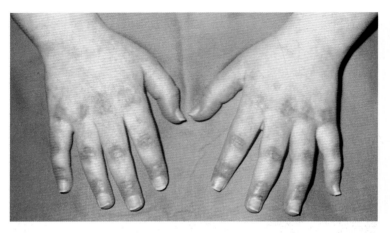

a) In what condition do these lesions occur and what are they called?

b) Name four other skin manifestations of this condition.

c) How is the diagnosis best confirmed?

Question 2.30

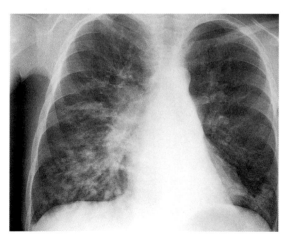

a) Name three abnormalities shown on this chest radiograph.

b) What condition most commonly gives this appearance?

Question 2.31

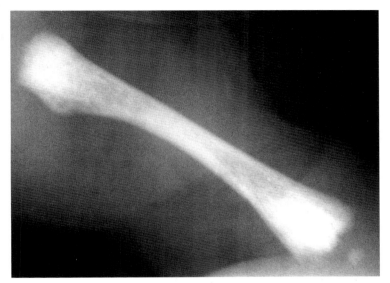

This newborn baby presented with growth retardation, rash and hepatosplenomegaly.

a) What is shown on this radiograph of the left femur?

b) What is the diagnosis?

Question 2.32

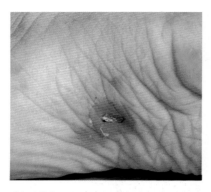

This three-year-old child presented with this single painful lesion on the dorsum of the foot.

a) What is the aetiology of this lesion?

Question 2.33

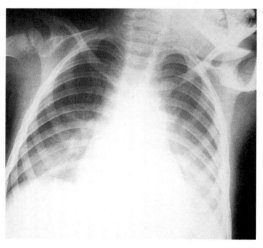

This eight-year old boy with known sickle cell disease presented with a two-day history of chest pain.

a) What complication of the disease is shown in this chest radiograph?

b) Name three important therapeutic interventions.

Question 2.34

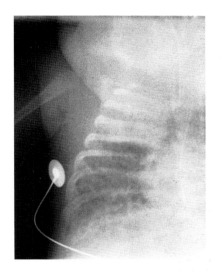

2

This chest radiograph is of a 14-week-old neonate, born at 24 weeks gestation, who remains oxygen and ventilator dependent.

a) What two complications are shown?

Question 2.35

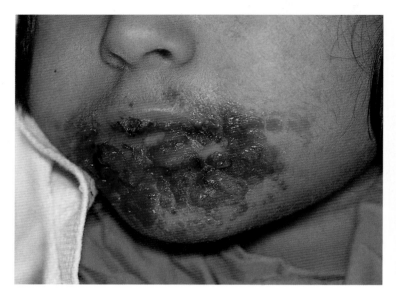

a) What is the name of this skin condition?

b) Name the two most commonly isolated organisms.

EXAM
QUESTIONS

1

2

3

4

5

6

Case History Paper

Question 3.1

A one-day-old male is referred from the postnatal ward with a history of inspiratory stridor. He was born at 39 weeks and weighed 8 lb 4 oz with an Apgar score of nine at one minute and ten at ten minutes. His mother is a 33-year-old primagravida who is rubella immune and VDRL negative and her blood group is O positive. The pregnancy was complicated by polyhydramnios, but ultrasound scanning did not report any abnormalities. The stridor is most marked when the child is supine. He is able to take a bottle without respiratory distress and appears otherwise well.

a) What two investigations are required?

b) Name two diagnoses that must be excluded.

Question 3.2

A six-week-old boy presents with repeated episodes of upper respiratory tract infection. He appears to be thriving, with his growth on the 50th centile for weight and head circumference. He has been started on 1% topical steroidal cream for eczema. His mother and father both have atopic histories.

The results of investigations are as follows:

- Hb   9 g/dl.
- WCC 6×10^9/l (lymphocytes 1×10^9/l, neutrophils 2×10^9/l, eosinophils 3×10^9/l).
- Platelet count 90×10^9/l.
- Direct Coombs' test   Positive.

a) What is the diagnosis?

Question 3.3

A two-year-old girl is referred to the outpatient clinic with a six-week history of a swelling in the right parotid region that has not responded to a prolonged course of amoxycillin. She has otherwise been well. She was born at term of Caucasian parents: dad works as a chauffeur and mother does part-time cleaning. There are no pets in the household.

She is up-to-date with her immunizations and has not travelled abroad. There is no history of any family illnesses. Her appetite is good, but she has a habit of eating soil. Her parents report no symptoms associated with this. There are no other siblings.

On examination she appears happy. She has a temperature of 37.5°C centrally and is on the 50th centile for height and weight. There are matted lesions within the right parotid region, which are not tender to touch. There is no associated bruit and there are no other similar masses. There is no hepatosplenomegaly and her other systems are normal.

a) What test should be performed?

b) Give a diagnosis.

Question 3.4

A 16-year-old girl presents with a one-day history of vomiting bright red blood. She has produced about 300 ml with effortless vomiting and appears pale. She has no past medical history apart from being on inhaled steroids for asthma, which was diagnosed six years ago. She has not travelled abroad, and does not smoke or drink.

She has two brothers – a third brother died at seven days of age from bowel obstruction. Her periods are irregular; she has no sexual history and her pubertal development appears delayed. She has not received any blood products and does not abuse drugs. Her parents are not related and there are no pets.

On examination she is clinically anaemic, clubbed and appears generally unwell. Her height is on the third centile, as is her weight. Her abdominal examination reveals hepatosplenomegaly with caput medusa. She also has glycosuria.

a) What is the diagnosis?

Question 3.5

A five-year-old Middle Eastern tourist arrived in the UK ten days before presentation and had been well until the previous evening when she became irritable, miserable and lethargic. She was pyrexial with a peripheral temperature of 39°C. She vomited twice and had ten episodes of watery green stool with large flecks of red blood. She has not had any antecedent features of upper respiratory tract infection, arthralgia or rash.

She was born by normal vaginal delivery at term. At four years of age she was admitted to hospital for adenoidectomy, which she underwent without any complications. She is not known to have any allergies and is up-to-date with her immunizations. Her family is Arabic, her mother being a 24-year-old housewife and her father a 36-year-old car mechanic. The parents are second cousins. There are no other children. They live in a village with electricity, but there have been problems with the water supply.

On examination her core temperature is 40°C, her heart rate 160 beats per minute and blood pressure 100/55 mm Hg in her right arm. Her capillary refill is over four seconds. Her chest is clear and her abdomen soft. Her Glasgow Coma Score is 10. There is no papilloedema, with a normal fundus being seen on fundoscopy and there is no focal neurology.

Results of initial investigations are:

- Hb   13.4 g/dl.
- WCC 3.5×10^9/l (lymphocytes 1×10^9/l, neutrophils 2×10^9/l, eosinophils 0.3×10^9/l).
- Platelet count 290×10^9/l.
- Sodium   124 mmol/l.
- Potassium   3.1 mmol/l.
- Urea   2.4 mmol/l.
- Creatinine   64 μmol/l
- Glucose   8 mmol/l.
- Albumin   32 g/l.
- Plasma osmolarity   272 mOsm/kg.
- PT   19.5 s (control 15 s).
- Ammonia   22 μmol/l.
- Bilirubin   26 μmol/l.
- Arterial blood gas   pH 7.44, bicarbonate 19 mmol/l, BE −4.
- Toxicology studies   Negative.

a) What are the three key clinical components?

b) Give two differential diagnoses.

Data Interpretation Paper

Question 3.6

A four-week-old boy presents with a three-day history of recurrent vomiting. The results of investigations are:

- Plasma sodium   137 mmol/l.
- Plasma potassium   3.4 mmol/l.
- Plasma chloride   83 mmol/l.
- Plasma urea   11 mmol/l.
- Plasma creatinine   60 μmol/l.
- Venous bicarbonate   41 mmol/l.
- Urinary pH   7.9.

a) Comment on these results.

b) What is the likely diagnosis?

Question 3.7

A six-week-old boy presents with failure to thrive, being off his feeds and having repeated bouts of vomiting. His blood pressure is 115/75 mm Hg in his right arm. The results of investigations are:

- Plasma sodium   129 mmol/l.
- Plasma potassium   7.8 mmol/l.
- Plasma chloride   97 mmol/l.
- Plasma urea   41 mmol/l.
- Plasma creatinine   360 μmol/l.
- Venous bicarbonate   13 mmol/l.
- Hb   6 g/dl.
- WCC 17×10^9/l.
- Platelet count 250×10^9/l.

a) How do you interpret these results?

Question 3.8

A four-year-old girl who is below the third centile for height and weight is otherwise well. Her heart rate is 90 beats per minute and she has a blood pressure of 90/55 mm Hg. The results of investigations are:

- Plasma sodium — 139 mmol/l.
- Plasma potassium — 2.2 mmol/l.
- Plasma chloride — 90 mmol/l.
- Plasma urea — 4.9 mmol/l.
- Plasma creatinine — 43 μmol/l.
- Venous bicarbonate — 33 mmol/l.

a) What is the diagnosis?

Question 3.9

A four-week-old boy presents with projectile vomiting. Results of investigations are:

- Plasma sodium — 128 mmol/l.
- Plasma potassium — 7.2 mmol/l.
- Plasma chloride — 99 mmol/l.
- Plasma urea — 10.9 mmol/l.
- Plasma creatinine — 83 μmol/l.
- Venous bicarbonate — 13 mmol/l.

a) What is the diagnosis and what is the mode of inheritance of this condition?

Question 3.10

A nine-month-old girl with marked diarrhoea and vomiting for two days has the following biochemical results:

- Plasma sodium — 173 mmol/l.
- Plasma potassium — 4.2 mmol/l.
- Plasma chloride — 132 mmol/l.
- Plasma urea — 2.9 mmol/l.
- Plasma creatinine — 103 μmol/l.
- Venous bicarbonate — 15 mmol/l.

a) What is the problem and how should she be managed?

Question 3.11

A three-day-old child suddenly collapses on the postnatal ward. His four limb blood pressures are as follows:

- Right arm   65/35 mm Hg.
- Left arm mean reading   20 mm Hg.
- Right leg mean reading   20 mm Hg.
- Left leg mean reading   20 mm Hg.

The results of his biochemistry are:

- Plasma sodium   153 mmol/l.
- Plasma potassium   4.2 mmol/l.
- Plasma chloride   102 mmol/l.
- Plasma urea   13.9 mmol/l.
- Plasma creatinine   83 μmol/l.
- Venous bicarbonate   15 mmol/l.
- Total calcium   0.9 mmol/l.

a) What is the cardiac abnormality?

b) What is the underlying condition?

Question 3.12

A boy can verbalize the need to go to the lavatory, put on his hat and shoes and has tantrums to gain attention.

a) How old is he?

Question 3.13

A 14-year-old boy is referred to outpatients as his general practitioner has found that he has microscopic haematuria. He also has bilateral sensorineural deafness and a younger brother is similarly affected.

a) What is the diagnosis?

Question 3.14

A five-year-old boy bleeds profusely after tonsillectomy. He has had episodes of recurrent nose bleeds. Preoperative results of blood tests are:

- Hb   7 g/dl.
- PCV   0.31.
- Platelets $300 \times 10^9/l$.

Results of further investigations postoperatively are:

- Bleeding time   20 minutes.
- PT   13 s (control 12 s).
- APTT   129 s (control 20 s).

a) What is the diagnosis?

Question 3.15

A seven-month-old girl has developed rickets despite a normal diet and has been taking vitamin D_2 (calciferol) 600 units per day and no other medications for the past three months. Her blood biochemistry is as follows:

- Calcium   2.01 mmol/l.
- Albumin   38 g/l.
- Phosphate   1.2 mmol/l (normal 1.3–1.9).
- Alkaline phosphatase 1235 IU/l.

a) What is the likely diagnosis?

Photographic Material Paper

Question 3.16

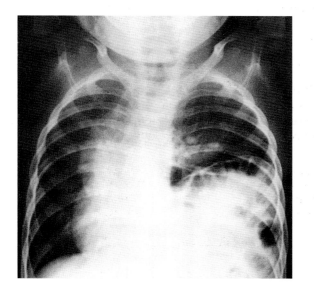

a) What is seen on this radiograph?

Question 3.17

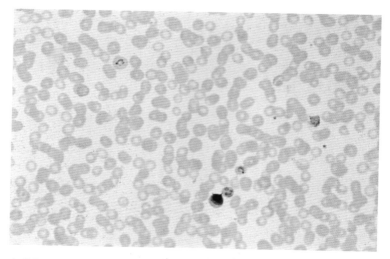

a) What is the diagnosis?

Question 3.18

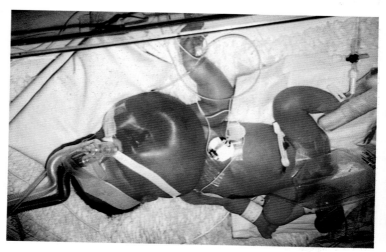

a) What is seen in the neck of this child?

b) What is the prognosis?

Question 3.19

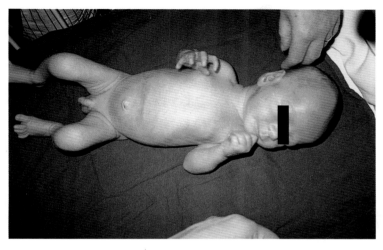

3

a) What operative procedure has this child had?

b) What was the underlying problem?

Question 3.20

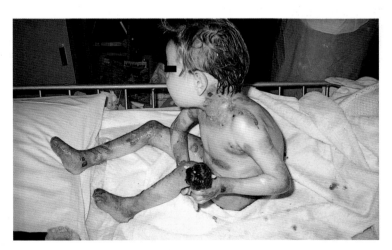

a) What is this child's condition?

b) What are the associated long-term complications?

Question 3.21

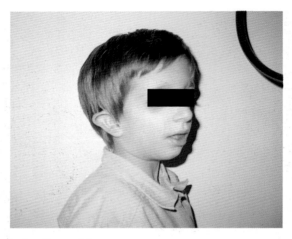

a) What is the diagnosis?

b) What are the associated anomalies?

Question 3.22

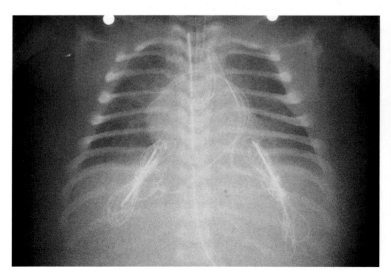

a) What is seen on this chest radiograph?

Question 3.23

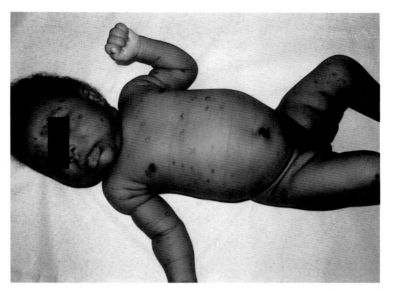

This is a six-week-old child who has a vesicular rash. The child had been well until the time this picture was taken.

a) What is the diagnosis?

b) Does the child need passive immunization?

Question 3.24

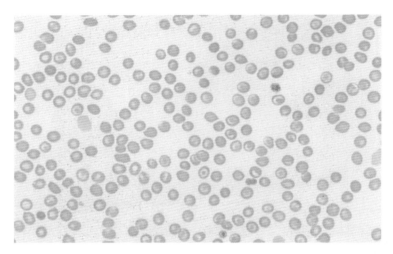

a) What abnormal cells are seen on this blood film?

Question 3.25

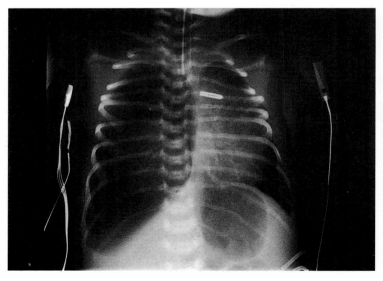

a) What are the main features of this chest radiograph?

Question 3.26

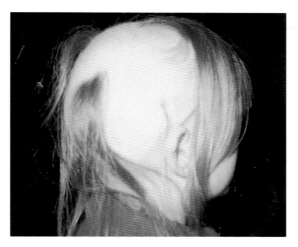

This girl was visiting her sister who was an inpatient with rheumatoid arthritis.

a) What is the association?

Question 3.27

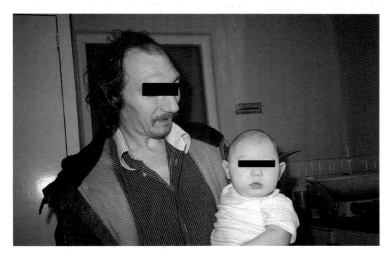

a) What is shown here?

Question 3.28

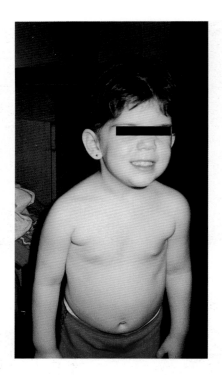

a) What is the diagnosis?

Question 3.29

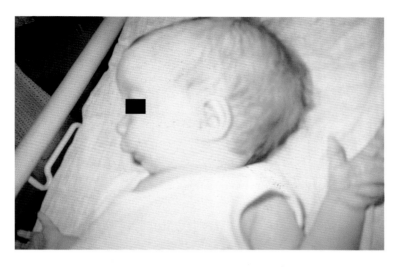

a) What are the associated features of this condition?

Question 3.30

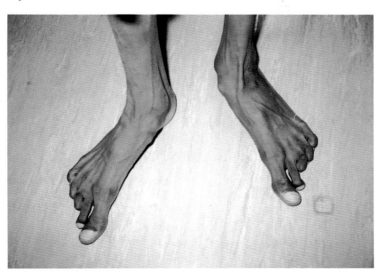

a) What is the diagnosis?

Question 3.31

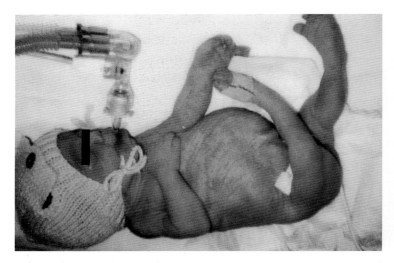

a) What is this condition?

Question 3.32

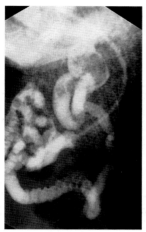

This preterm neonate developed necrotizing enterocolitis requiring a defunctioning ileostomy. Before reanastomosis a barium contrast study was performed through the distal limb of the stoma.

a) What is seen?

Question 3.33

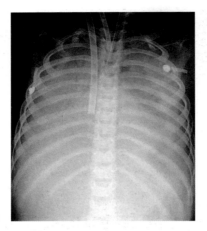

a) What treatment is this patient receiving?

Question 3.34

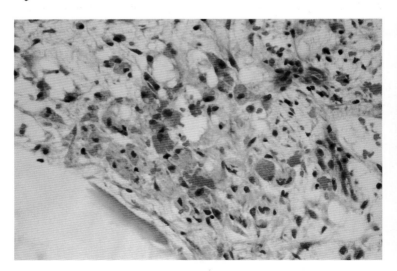

This is the bone marrow of an infant who presented with hepato-splenomegaly and failure to thrive.

a) What is the diagnosis?

Question 3.35

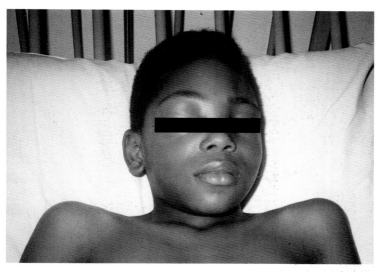

3

a) What complication can arise in this patient with orbital cellulitis?

EXAM
QUESTIONS

1
2
3
4
5
6

Case History Paper

Question 4.1

A three-year-old boy is brought to the accident and emergency department with a left-sided facial palsy. He has been generally unwell over the past month and has been losing weight and his appetite is poor. He looks pale and is quiet. He was born at term by vaginal delivery and had until this episode been well. He is up-to-date with his immunizations. His mother is a single parent and there are no other children. Dad is working abroad and has not been back to the UK since his son was born. The boy has not travelled abroad. He does not have any known allergies.

On examination he is listless and his Glasgow Coma Score is about 13. He has a left-sided facial palsy and is noted to have a right-sided hemi-hypertrophy. There is no cervical lympadenopathy and no clubbing, but he appears anaemic. Examination of his cardiovascular system reveals a flow murmur at the left sternal border and a heart rate of 100 beats per minute. His blood pressure in his right arm is 156/99 mm Hg. His chest is clear. His abdomen is distended with a 3 cm palpable liver edge displaced by a mass 10 cm by 14 cm. There is no bruit to the mass, but it is not possible to palpate underneath the mass. An abdominal radiograph is normal, but an abdominal ultrasound shows a suprarenal mass on the right.

a) What are the priorites in this boy's treatment?

b) What two investigations should be performed?

Question 4.2

A 13-year-old male who has been excluded from school for temper tantrums and ill-discipline is referred to the paediatric outpatients by the school doctor. He has had recurrent episodes of central abdominal pain. An ultrasound examination shows stippling of the right and left kidneys. His blood pressure at initial attendance to the clinic is 145/95 mm Hg, but when repeated in the examination room is 100/70 mm Hg.

a) What is the diagnois?

b) What complications have arisen?

Question 4.3

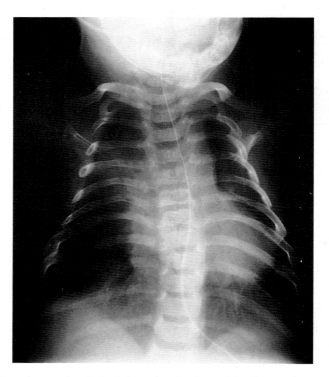

A 38-week-gestation baby is born by elective epidural caesarian section as the two previous deliveries were also delivered in this manner. Mother is a social worker and father is a law student, aged 23 and 25, respectively. They are not related and do not have any past medical history of note. The pregnancy has been normal and the scan at 11 weeks confirmed the date of gestation based on the last menstrual period. Apgar scores at one and five minutes are nine and ten, respectively, with minimal intervention required apart from drying the baby. He is noticed to have a reduced thoracic diameter and has some respiratory difficulty. He is very small for his age and requires headbox oxygen for six weeks. All septic screens performed are negative. Repeated testing for immunodeficiency states, cystic fibrosis and Schwachmann syndrome is negative.

a) Comment on his chest radiograph shown above.

b) What is the diagnosis?

Question 4.4

The following is taken from a referral letter to a hepatologist. 'Thank you for seeing this six-week-old boy who was born by normal vaginal delivery with normal scores. His birth weight was 2.9 kg and his occipitofrontal circumference was 33 cm. He received phototherapy on day 2 of life for 48 hours. An abdominal ultrasound showed a normal gall bladder and common bile duct and there was no evidence of a choleduochal cyst. He was discharged home on day 7. His mother is a 22-year-old primigravida. There is no family history of note. At three weeks he was still noticed to be jaundiced.'

Results of investigations so far are:

- Hb   10.4 g/dl.
- WCC $5.5 \times 10^9/1$.
- Platelet count $390 \times 10^9/1$.
- Haptoglobins   Normal levels.
- Fibrinogen products   Normal levels.
- Sodium   144 mmol/l.
- Potassium   4.1 mmol/l.
- Urea   4.4 mmol/l.
- Creatinine   64 μmol/l.
- Glucose   8 mmol/l.
- Albumin   39 g/l.
- γ glutamyl transferase   472 IU/l.
- Alanine transferase   55 IU/l.
- Alkaline phosphatase   162 IU/l.
- PT   19.5 s (control 15 s).
- Bilirubin   199 μmol/l.
- Conjugated bilirubin   7 μmol/l.
- Venous blood gas pH   7.28.
- Urine reducing substances   Negative.
- Blood cultures and urine cultures   Negative.
- α-1-antitrypsin phenotype   Normal.
- Hepatitis A and B serology   Negative.
- Serology for TORCH and syphilis   Normal.
- Immunoreactive trypsin levels   Normal.

On examination at his three-week outpatient appointment he appears deeply jaundiced, pale and lethargic. His stools are coloured and his urine is yellow. He has a firm 3 cm liver. No other masses are palpable. Other systems are normal apart from generalized hypotonia, a small penis and pale discs on fundoscopy.

a) What is the diagnosis?

Question 4.5

The following copy is taken from a referral letter to a retrieval team picking up a baby for intensive care for respiratory distress. 'Thank you for taking this infant who was born at term at which time she weighed 8 lb. She was breastfed for three days and then fed with formula feeds. She was admitted with RSV positive bronchiolitis at the age of two months, but was discharged the following day as she was only mildly affected. She returned 14 days later with marked respiratory distress, requiring 60% oxygen delivered via a headbox. A chest radiograph showed widespread opacifications throughout both lung fields. FBC showed her Hb to be 5 g/dl with a neutropenia and low platelets. She was topped up and continued on intravenous cefotaxime and gradually improved.

There was no evidence of haemolysis on her blood film and she was direct Coombs' test negative. Her G6PD, liver function tests, calcium, creatinine, CRP, ESR, calcium, urea and creatinine are all within normal limits. PCR for HIV and culture are negative as is antibody testing for HIV. She is of Asian origin and the parents are first cousins and she is their first child.

The current picure is of respiratory distress with arterial blood gases showing a pH of 7.42, P_{CO_2} 9.6 kPa, P_{O_2} 6.1 kPa, BE 4.6. She has a peripheral O_2 saturation reading of 85% and marked respiratory distress. She is tachycardiac at 150 beats per minute with a capillary refill time of two seconds and her blood pressure in the right arm is 80/50 mm Hg. Her chest has marked bilateral crackles with tracheal tug and air hunger. She is alert and her pupils equal and reactive. There is no focal neurological deficit. She also has broadened thumbs, large toes, a high arched palate, microcephaly and short stature. She has patches of eczematous areas on her arms and legs and café au lait patches on her trunk, but there is no organomegaly. She has a harsh pansystolic murmur best heard at the left sternal edge.

A bone marrow examination has revealed a hypocellular marrow. Today's chest radiograph shows widespread pulmonary infiltates and the presence of a thymus. There is also an enlarged heart, which has a boot shape.'

a) What is the diagnosis?

Data Interpretation Paper

Question 4.6

A 14-month-old Caucasian boy is admitted with dehydration and the following blood test results:

- Plasma sodium 127 mmol/l.
- Plasma potassium 2.7 mmol/l.
- Plasma chloride 87 mmol/l.
- Plasma urea 6.6 mmol/l.
- Plasma creatinine 32 μmol/l.
- Venous bicarbonate 41 mmol/l.
- Urinary sodium 7.9 mmol/l.
- Plasma pH 7.49.
- Plasma aldosterone 1100 pmol/l (normal range 60–900 pmol/l).
- Sweat sodium 70 mmol/l.

His blood pressure is 90/75 mm Hg and he is due to attend the outpatient clinic for investigation of failure to thrive.

a) What is the diagnosis?

Question 4.7

A ten-year-old boy presents to casualty apparently inebriated, with a metabolic acidosis and an increased anion gap. Ethanol is not detected on blood analysis. His BM stix is 6 mmol/l.

a) How do you account for this picture?

Question 4.8

You are asked to see a neonate who has ambiguous genitalia with one gonad palpable in the inguinal canal. Blood 17-hydroxyprogesterone levels are elevated and ultrasound of the abdomen shows internal female organs. Chromosomal analysis reveals 46 XX karyotype.

a) What two tests should be performed?

Question 4.9

An eight-month-old boy is admitted with failure to thrive. He is hirsute, but appears otherwise normal. His medication initially was captopril, but has included minoxidil for the past four months. His chest radiograph shows cardiomegaly and an ECG reveals left ventricular hypertrophy, with an ejection fraction of 46% (normal is greater than 60%). He has not had any instrumentation of his umbilical vessels. His renal ultrasound shows normal size kidneys, which have a normal echogenic pattern. His abdominal vessels are thought to be small for his age. Five days after his admission he develops a sudden rise in his blood pressure as a gradual withdrawal in his hypertensive control has been attempted. The blood pressure in his right arm increases from 97–114/47–67 mm Hg to 150–160/90 mm Hg. This is associated with hepatomegaly and respiratory distress and he is intubated and ventilated. Repeated urine cultures have been negative and biochemical analysis of his urine has been unremarkable. His renal function is within normal limits as is his DMSA and MCUG. His plasma renin levels are grossly elevated.

Arterial catheterization is performed and the results are as follows.

	Systolic pressure (mm Hg)	Diastolic pressure (mm Hg)
Ascending aorta	107	55
Descending aorta	102	55
Pulmonary artery	16	4

His four limb blood pressures are:

- Left arm   100/50 mm Hg.
- Right arm   100/50 mm Hg.
- Left leg   100/50 mm Hg.
- Right leg   100/50 mm Hg.

a) What is the diagnosis?

Question 4.10

There is a visual field defect of a bitemporal hemianopia in a six-year-old girl. She complains of frequent recurrent headaches.

a) Where is the possible site of disturbance to the visual pathways?

b) What could this lesion be due to?

Question 4.11

A 12-year-old girl has recurrent episodes of facial swelling. The following complement studies are performed while she is having an attack:

- C2   Low.
- CH50   Low.
- C3   Normal.
- C4   Low.

a) What is the most likely diagnosis?

Question 4.12

 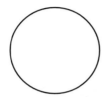 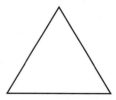

a) With what age would these drawings be compatible?

Question 4.13

A six-month-old child is admitted with a history of easy bruising and frequent nose bleeds. Results of investigations are:

- Hb   9.6 g/dl.
- WCC $8 \times 10^9/l.$
- Platelet count $36 \times 10^9/l.$
- Blood film   Normal apart from showing large sized platelets.
- PT   1.1 ratio.
- APPT   Normal.
- von Willebrand's factor Normal limits.
- Platelet aggregation   Defective with ristocetin, but normal with ADP, adrenaline and collagen.

a) What is this condition?

Question 4.14

	O₂ Saturation (%)	Pressure (mm Hg)
Superior vena cava	76	6
Inferior vena cava	74	6
Right atrium	84	7
Right ventricle	85	20/7
Pulmonary artery	85	20/13
Left atrium	97	8
Left ventricle	96	121/75–7
Aorta	97	129/75

a) Interpret the cardiac catheter data given above and give a diagnosis.

Question 4.15

A one-week-old child presents with a shrill cry and general irritability. A septic screen is clear, but urinary amino acids reveal a high concentration of valine, isoleucine and leucine.

a) What is the diagnosis?

Photographic Material Paper

Question 4.16

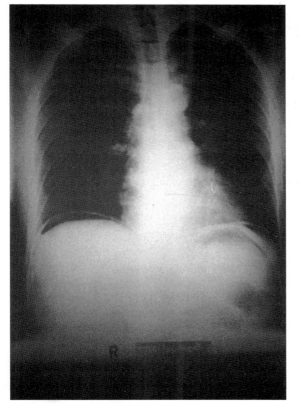

a) What is the abnormality on this radiograph?

Question 4.17

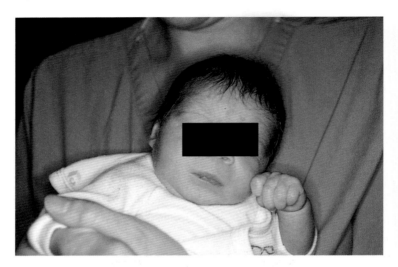

This child has an ASD and initially presented with failure to thrive.

a) What syndrome does this child have?

Question 4.18

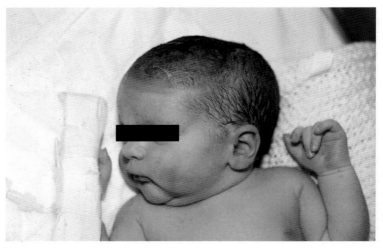

a) What has happened to this neonate?

Question 4.19

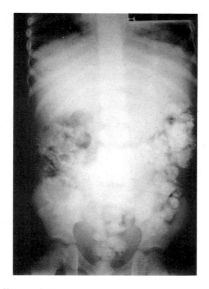

a) What is the diagnosis?

Question 4.20

4

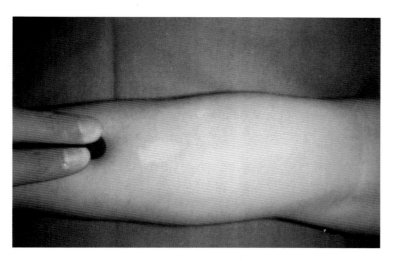

a) What is this lesion?

Question 4.21

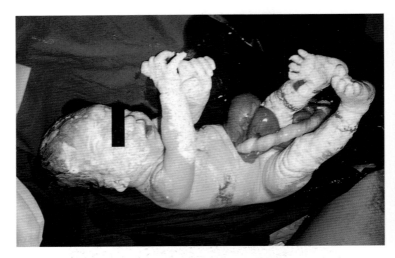

a) What is this condition?

Question 4.22

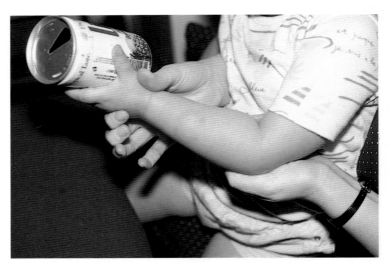

a) What is seen on this child's arm?

Question 4.23

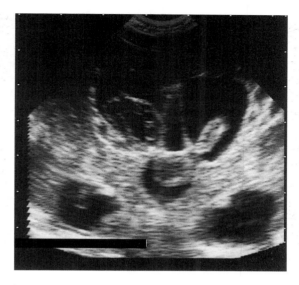

a) What is seen in this ultrasound study of an unwell neonate?

Question 4.24

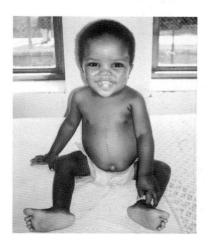

This child has sparse reddish hair and a prominent forehead.

a) What is the matter with this child?

Question 4.25

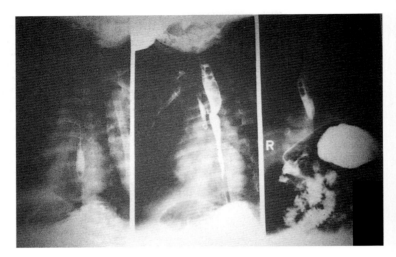

a) What does this study show?

Question 4.26

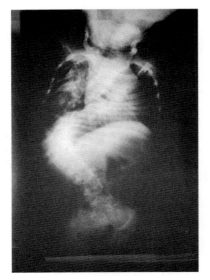

a) What is seen on this radiograph?

Question 4.27

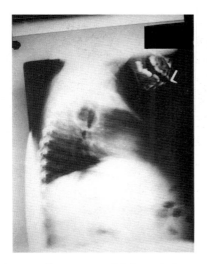

a) What is the abnormality seen on this lateral chest radiograph?

Question 4.28

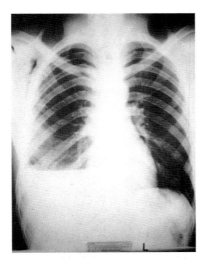

4

a) What does this child who has been involved in a road traffic accident have?

Question 4.29

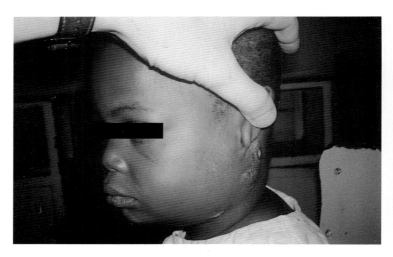

These lesions are not warm, but are firm to touch.

a) What are they due to?

Question 4.30

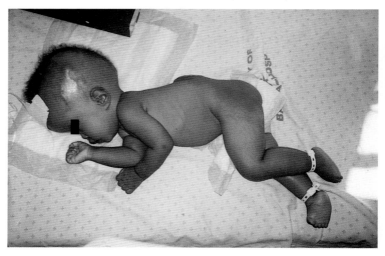

a) What is seen in this child?

Question 4.31

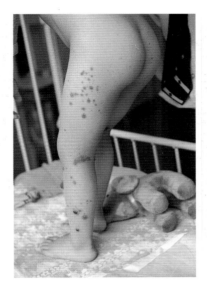

This child has haematuria and abdominal pain.

a) What condition does he have?

4

Question 4.32

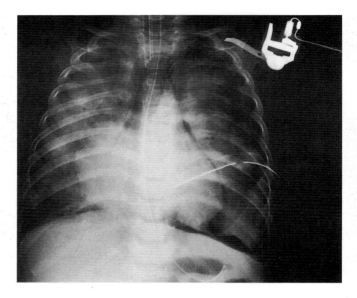

a) What is seen on this radiograph?

Question 4.33

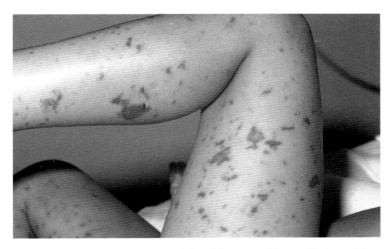

This child is disorientated, pyrexial and has a capillary refill time of four seconds.

a) What does this slide show?

b) What is the diagnosis?

Question 4.34

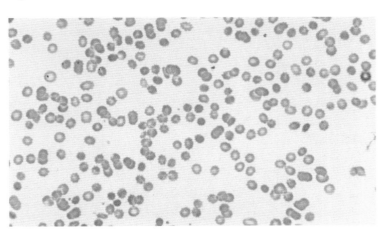

a) What are the abnormal cells seen in this picture?

Question 4.35

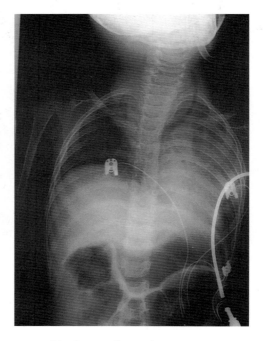

a) What is seen on this chest radiograph?

EXAM
QUESTIONS

1
2
3
4
5
6

Case History Paper

Question 5.1

A nine-year-old girl is referred by the school doctor for assessment of her growth. The girl was the tallest in the class (height 154.1 cm; weight 57.5 kg) and had been so for some time. She has been teased by her classmates, particularly as she has marked facial acne. The school doctor has noted the presence of pubic hair, which had been present for some time according to the girl's mother. She has not begun her menses. There is no significant past history although she suffered a trivial head injury three years previously requiring an overnight hospital admission. A skull radiograph had been normal although her mother was fairly convinced that her daughter had been concussed. She has one sister of 22 months. Her mother is an accountant with a gynaecological history of subfertility. This had necessitated the use of clomiphene treatment. Father is a teacher. He can remember being taken to see a paediatrician regarding his growth when a child.

Examination reveals advanced puberty (B1 P3 A2). There is abundant pubic and axillary hair, but no breast development. Clitoromegaly is noted. An acneiform skin rash is particularly florid over the scapula region. There are no other skin lesions. Her blood pressure is 110/60 mm Hg.

The following results of investigations were obtained:

- Bone age   15.2 years.
- Hb   12.1 g/dl.
- Sodium   141 mmol/l.
- Potassium   4.6 mmol/l.
- Urea   3.1 mmol/l.
- T_4 80 nmol/l (normal 65–160).
- TSH   0.61 mU/l (normal 0.25–6).
- Cortisol 09.00   350 nmol/l (normal 140–690).
- Cortisol 24.00   140 nmol/l.
- ACTH   68 ng/l (normal 10–45).
- FSH   2 IU/l.
- Androstenedione   34.8 nmol/l (normal 2–12).

5

a) Give three useful investigations to aid diagnosis.

b) What is the most likely diagnosis?

c) Outline 3 components of the treatment plan.

Question 5.2

A 12-year-old Filipino boy is admitted with a febrile illness, which he has had for the preceding nine days. The fever had commenced abruptly and had regularly been measured at 39.8°C orally by his mother. He had developed knee pain and a sore throat. On the day of admission, an erythematous rash had appeared over his feet and extensor surfaces of his upper limbs. There were areas of petechiae and purpura over his elbows. While nauseated, he had not vomited, although he was passing the occasional diarrhoeal stool.

At four years of age he had undergone a tonsillectomy and at six years of age he suffered viral meningitis. He had had the usual number of upper respiratory tract infections for his age, but no further serious illnesses. He has a 15-year-old brother who was diagnosed as diabetic two years ago. There has been no recent foreign travel and the family do not have any pets.

On examination he looks unwell and is febrile with a temperature of 40°C. There is clinically no obvious focus for his fever. His tongue is coated and his lips are cracked. A fine petechial rash covers his elbows and purpura are superimposed on his marked erythema multiforme over his lower limbs. Hepatosplenomegaly is noted, together with discrete anterior triangle cervical lymphadenopathy. He is normotensive and well perfused, with a capillary refill time of two seconds. There is no evidence of nuchal rigidity, and although conscious he is notably disorientated. Severe oral ulceration is noted.

The following test results are obtained:

- Hb   8.9 g/dl.
- WCC 1.2×10^9/l. (neutrophils 20%).
- Platelets 53×10^9/l.
- ESR   89 mm/h.
- Sodium   133 mmol/l.
- Potassium   3.5 mmol/l.
- Urea   10.2 mmol/l.
- Creatinine   146 μmol/l.
- Urinalysis   Proteinuria +++, haematuria ++.
- Septic screen   Sterile including CSF and blood.

- CRP   4 mg/l.
- Anti-streptolysin O titre (ASOT) Less than 200 IU/l.
- C4   0.05 IU/l (normal 0.2–1.7).
- C3   0.34 IU/l (normal 0.7–3.4).
- Viral serology for adenovirus,
  cytomegalovirus, herpes simplex,
  Epstein–Barr virus and
  human herpes type 6   Negative
- Mycoplasma IgM   Negative

a) Give three further investigations to aid diagnosis.

b) What is the most likely diagnosis?

c) Give two appropriate treatments for your diagnosis.

Question 5.3

The neonatal team is crash called to the delivery suite. A 33-week gestation infant had been born in poor condition following an emergency caesarean section performed for profound fetal bradycardia and associated passage of meconium. Mother had attended the clinic as she had felt diminished fetal movements over the last 48 hours.

On examination, the infant, weighing 2 kg, is blue and gasping. The heart rate is 80/min. The neonatal registrar intubates the baby with a 3.0 mm oral endotracheal tube and commences ventilation. There is no evidence of meconium below the vocal cords. There is an improvement in heart rate, but the infant remains poorly responsive and hypotonic with little respiratory effort. During resuscitation, widespread petechiae are noted. The infant is transferred to the neonatal intensive care unit at 15 minutes of age. A sudden deterioration occurs immediately after transfer. A massive pulmonary haemorrhage is noted and necessitates both reintubation and increased mechanical ventilation settings. Despite multisystem support, the infant becomes steadily more hypotensive and suffers an asystolic cardiac arrest, which is unresponsive to therapy.

Mother is a 34-year-old barrister. This is her second child. Her pregnancy has been unremarkable, with normal ultrasound scans. She suffered an acute bout of chest pain four days before the delivery of her baby. This chest pain had necessitated the use of dihydrocodeine for pain relief. However, she was well on the day of delivery.

The results of investigations performed on the baby include:

- Hb   12.4 g/dl.
- WCC 2.1×10^9/l.

- Platelets $54 \times 10^9/l.$
- PT   42 s.
- APTT   56 s.
- FDPs   Elevated.
- Blood culture   No growth.
- Urine culture   No growth.
- Maternal HVS   No growth.
- CSF examination   Red cells $950/mm^3$, white cells $19/mm^3$, (predominantly lymphocytes), glucose 4.2 mmol/l, protein 0.9 g/l, culture – no growth.
- Chest radiograph   Complete 'white out' with a pneumo-mediastinum.

a) What is the diagnosis?

b) What is the probable aetiological agent in this case?

c) What is the treatment?

Question 5.4

An 11-year-old boy is referred to the outpatient clinic with a six-week history of intermittent fever, periumbilical pain, frequent headaches and a subjective sense of cold. He was previously well. The family had been on holiday to Malta three months ago. He has a twin brother and an older sister who are asymptomatic. All the symptoms began abruptly following a minor illness lasting 48 hours associated with nausea, fever and loose stools.

Examination is unremarkable, but he is admitted for further investigation. Despite subjective feelings to the contrary, no fever can be documented. He is very tearful when his mother leaves his bedside. Three days after admission, he complains of blurred vision and dizziness. He feels weak and requires two nurses to help him to the toilet.

Mother is a teacher and father has his own garage. There is a family history of rheumatoid arthritis. His maternal uncle died 11 months earlier following a road traffic accident. He is an intelligent school boy who has recently sat and passed an entrance examination for a local school. He is usually top of the class, but has not attended school for the last few weeks as he is in pain and too tired.

Results of the investigations are as follows:

- Hb   13.4 g/dl.
- Blood film   Normal.

- Monospot   Negative.
- ESR   3 mm/h.
- Liver function tests   Normal.
- TSH   2.5 mU/l.
- Rheumatoid factor   Negative.
- Antinuclear antibody   Negative.
- Anti-smooth muscle antibody   Weakly positive.
- Septic screen including stool culture   No growth.
- Epstein–Barr virus serology   Negative.
- Enteroviral IgM   Positive.
- MRI cranial scan   Normal.

Despite discharge home, readmittance is necessary two weeks later as he can no longer stand. His symptoms are still present, but he now complains of an inability to hear. An audiogram is normal. He also complains of deteriorating vision despite normal visual acuity testing. Repeat blood tests are normal.

a) What is the most likely unifying diagnosis?

b) What is the proposed pathophysiology?

c) Outline your therapeutic approach.

Question 5.5

A 34-week gestation infant is admitted to neonatal intensive care with respiratory distress. Mother is 29 years of age and this is her first pregnancy. She had suffered a threatened miscarriage at nine-weeks' gestation. Subsequently, serial ultrasound scans had demonstrated a symmetrically growth-retarded fetus. A maternal α-fetoprotein estimation had been double the normal, but this had been explained by the threatened miscarriage.

The infant requires a maximum FiO_2 of 0.55 in headbox only. His chest radiograph is considered to be consistent with transient tachypnoea of the newborn. An umbilical line is sited, but removed following radiography as it is a venous rather than arterial line. He begins to become steadily oedematous over the next 72 hours despite improvement in his respiratory function. Although severely oedematous, his general examination is normal with the exception of bilaterally undescended testes and perineal hypospadias. Results of investigations are as follows:

- Hb   8.5 g/dl.
- Platelets 35×10^9/l.
- Creatinine   76 μmol/l.
- Sodium   121 mmol/l.

- Potassium   3.2 mmol/l.
- Urea   7.8 mmol/l.
- Albumin   9 g/l.
- Liver function tests   Normal.
- Septic screen   No growth.
- Cranial ultrasound   Normal.
- ECG   Normal.
- Echocardiogram   Normal.
- Abdominal radiograph   Ascites.

a) List three other useful investigations to aid diagnosis.

b) What is the most likely diagnosis?

c) What is the association with the abnormal perineal examination?

Data Interpretation Paper

Question 5.6

A seven-year-old girl is noted to have a painless goitre on routine examination. She is clinically euthyroid. Thyroid function tests reveal:

- TSH   Less than 0.1 mU/l.
- T_4 109 nmol/l (normal 65–160).
- T_3 12.9 pmol/l (normal 4.3–9.2).
- ESR   5 mm/h.
- Hb   12.3 g/dl.

a) List two further helpful investigations.

b) What is the most likely diagnosis?

c) What is the natural history of the disorder?

Question 5.7

A five-year-old girl presents with tall stature. Examination is normal although she displays signs of pubertal development. There are no café au lait patches. She is euthyroid. Investigations are as follows:

- Tanner staging   B3 P3 A1.
- Skeletal bone age   8.8 years.
- 17-ß oestradiol   0.17 nmol/l.

The GnRH (LHRH) test provides the following information:

Time (min)	LH (IU/l)	FSH (IU/l)
0	4	6
30	102	28
60	77	26
90	49	25
120	42	25

a) What is the cause of her tall stature?

b) Explain the above results.

c) Outline your treatment of this disorder.

Question 5.8

A three-week-old infant, born at 32 weeks' gestation, develops profound apnoeic episodes. These are unrelated to feeds and are unresponsive to caffeine administration. She is noted to be febrile and increasingly irritable. A septic screen is performed. Results of investigations are as follows:

- Hb   9.8 g/dl.
- WCC 11×10^9/l.
- Platelets 115×10^9/l.
- Glucose   10.4 mmol/l.
- Sodium   118 mmol/l.
- Potassium   6.0 mmol/l.
- Urea   3.2 mmol/l.
- CRP   16 mg/l.
- Urine (bag)   50 WBCs and scanty organisms on microscopy.

a) What other test is indicated immediately?

b) List four other useful investigations.

c) What is the most likely diagnosis?

Question 5.9

A baby is born to a mother with a previous history of hepatitis B infection. The maternal serological status is:

- HBsAg   Positive.
- HBeAg   Negative.
- HBeAb   Positive.
- HBanti-cAg IgG   Positive.

a) Explain the above serological pattern.

b) What is the appropriate management of the newborn baby?

Question 5.10

A 13-year-old girl is referred with asymptomatic hepatomegaly, noted on routine school examination. Inflammatory bowel disease had been diagnosed two years previously, but her symptoms have been easily controlled by mesalazine. The following results are obtained:

- Bilirubin   8 μmol/l.
- Alanine transaminase   350 IU/l.
- Alkaline phosphatase   145 IU/l.
- INR   1.1.
- Hb   11.2 g/dl.
- ESR   75 mm/h.
- Antinuclear antibody (ANA)   Positive.
- Antimitochondrial antibody   Positive.

a) List two potential diagnoses.

b) List two tests to confirm the diagnosis.

c) What is the treatment?

Question 5.11

The following arterial blood gas was taken from a 27-week gestation infant weighing 790 g, who deteriorated during intermittent mandatory ventilation.

- pH   7.22.
- Po_2 5.4 kPa.
- Pco_2 7.9 kPa.
- BE   −4.
- Bicarbonate 17 mmol/l.

a) List three possible causes for the above results.

b) List four actions that could be performed to aid diagnosis.

c) List two ventilatory manipulations that may ameliorate this blood gas result.

Question 5.12

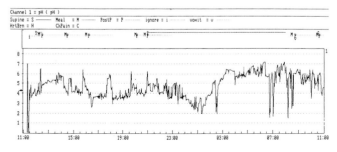

a) What is this investigation?

b) What does this investigation identify?

c) What is the appropriate management?

Question 5.13

A two-year-old boy returns from holiday with secondarily infected varicella. He is well with evidence of healing varicella lesions. The following biochemical results are obtained:

- Bilirubin   5 μmol/l.
- ALT   17 IU/l.

- Alkaline phosphatase   3369 IU/l. Isoenzymes. Predominantly bone.
- CRP   4 mg/l.
- Hb   11.3 g/dl.
- WCC $7.4 \times 10^9/l$.
- ESR   9 mm/h.

a) What is the likely diagnosis?

b) What is the treatment?

Question 5.14

A 12-year-old is admitted with intermittently painful fingertips. This developed three days after a prolonged respiratory tract infection. Her radial and ulnar pulses are normal, but the tips of her fingers are cold and slightly cyanosed. There is no central cyanosis. The signs and symptoms are exacerbated when her hands are placed in cold water. Investigations reveal:

- Hb   9 g/dl.
- WCC $8.2 \times 10^9/l$.
- Platelets $479 \times 10^9/l$.
- ESR   78 mm/h.
- CRP   32 mg/l.
- Blood film   Rouleaux.

a) Give two investigations to aid diagnosis.

b) What is the most likely diagnosis?

c) List four other complications of this disease.

Question 5.15

A three-week-old baby born normally at term, is admitted following a seizure. A full septic screen is normal. A cranial ultrasound scan is normal. Routine biochemical analysis is normal. There is marked improvement when feeds are discontinued. After a period of intravenous fluids and observation, feeds are restarted. The baby has another seizure associated with apnoea. Further evaluation reveals:

- Glucose   11.2 mmol/l.
- Sodium   134 mmol/l.
- Calcium   2.3 mmol/l.
- Phosphate   1.7 mmol/l.
- Urinary amino acids   Excess of isoleucine, leucine and valine.

a) What is the diagnosis?

b) What is the management?

Photographic Material Paper

Question 5.16

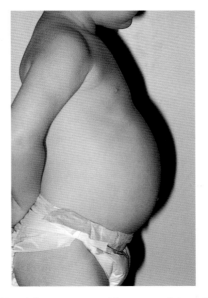

This two-year-old toddler presents with poor weight gain together with the passage of loose pungent stools. There is no organomegaly.

a) List four differential diagnoses.

b) List four important investigations to aid diagnosis.

Question 5.17

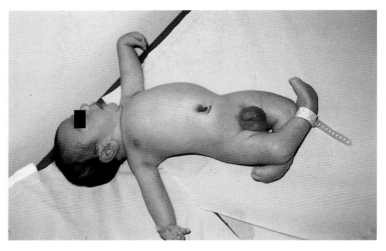

This newborn baby was delivered after the mother complained of decreased fetal movements. There are no apparent bony abnormalities.

a) What is the most likely diagnosis?

b) List four useful investigations to uncover the underlying aetiology.

c) What is the likely prognosis?

Question 5.18

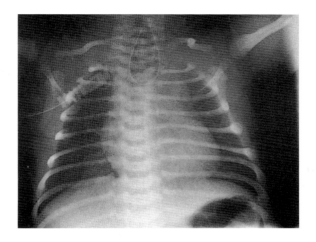

a) What is the diagnosis?

b) Why is this baby at risk of developing respiratory symptoms?

c) What clue would have been apparent in the antenatal period?

5

Question 5.19

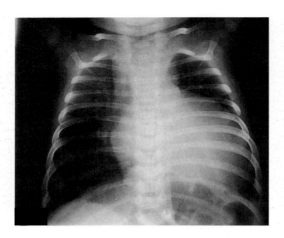

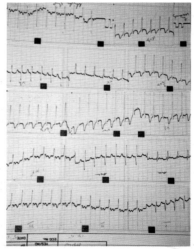

The above chest radiograph and ECG were obtained from a three-month-old infant who presented with failure to thrive and tachypnoea.

a) What does the chest radiograph show?

b) What does the ECG show?

c) What is the diagnosis?

d) Why was the baby tachypnoeic?

Question 5.20

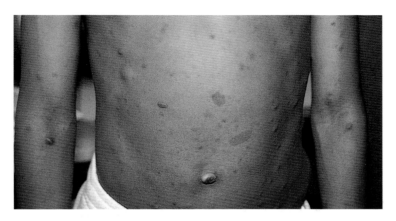

a) What is shown in this picture?

b) List four other features of this disorder.

c) Outline the long-term management.

Question 5.21

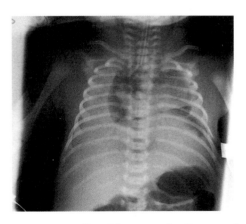

5

A preterm neonate was ventilated for severe hyaline membrane disease. A chest radiograph was obtained because of deteriorating respiratory function.

a) What is shown on this radiograph?

b) What is the management?

Question 5.22

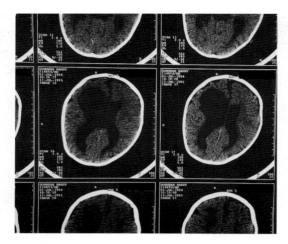

A nine-month-old boy is referred for neurodevelopmental assessment of a left hemiparesis. He was born at 29 weeks' gestation and required ventilation for four days due to hyaline membrane disease.

a) What is the above investigation?

b) What does it show?

c) What is the probable antecedent neonatal history?

Question 5.23

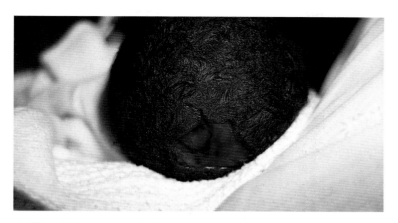

a) What is demonstrated above?

b) Give two possible aetiological diagnoses.

c) List three further investigations to help with diagnosis.

Question 5.24

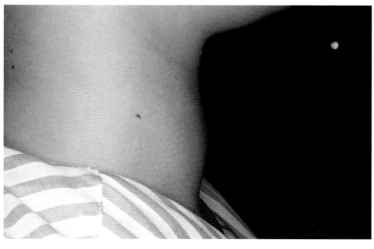

5

a) What is the diagnosis?

b) List three further useful investigations.

Question 5.25

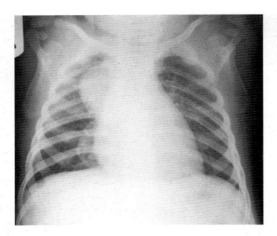

A six-month-old girl presented with a one-month history of wheezing. This chest radiograph was obtained.

a) Describe the above appearance.

b) What is the most likely diagnosis?

c) Give three further useful investigations.

d) What is the likely prognosis?

Question 5.26

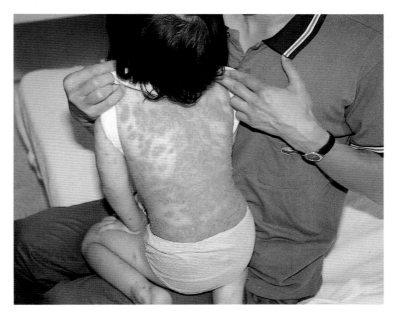

This girl is mildly systemically unwell.

a) What is the diagnosis?

b) What is the treatment?

5

Question 5.27

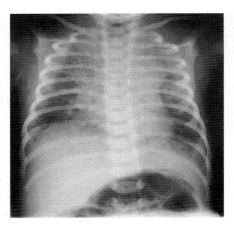

This infant was born at 42 weeks' gestation following prolonged abnormalities on the cardiotocograph.

a) What is the most likely diagnosis?

b) What is the pathophysiology accounting for the subsequent respiratory distress?

c) Outline your management of this case.

Question 5.28

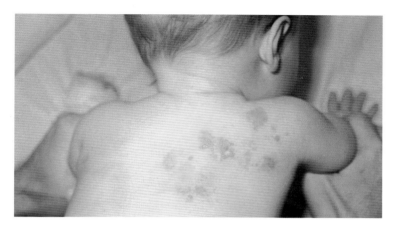

A 22-month-old infant is admitted with irritability. She has a low-grade fever without an obvious focus. She has recently finished chemotherapy for acute lymphoblastic leukaemia.

a) What is the diagnosis?

b) What is your management?

Question 5.29

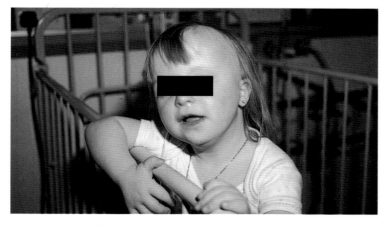

a) What is the diagnosis?

b) List four other chronic complications of the underlying diagnosis.

Question 5.30

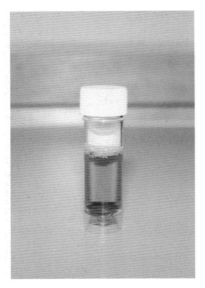

The above clinical sample is obtained from a four-week-old baby born at term who is jaundiced.

a) What is demonstrated?

b) List six investigations to aid diagnosis.

c) What colour are the stools most likely to be?

Question 5.31

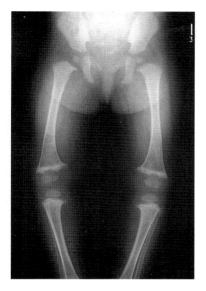

A 14-month-old Asian baby is referred with delayed milestones. The infant has not crawled or stood. The baby's mother had suffered from postnatal depression. The baby is still exclusively breast fed. This radiograph is obtained.

a) Give three abnormal radiological features.

b) What is the diagnosis?

c) What is the treatment?

5

Question 5.32

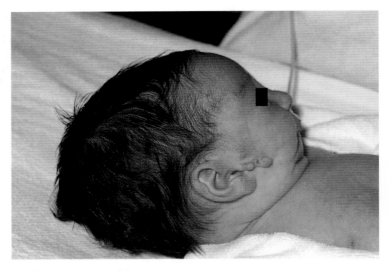

a) What is the most likely diagnosis?

b) Give three other features associated with this diagnosis.

Question 5.33

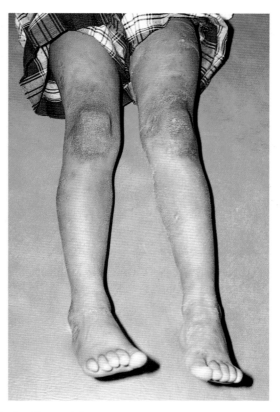

a) What is the diagnosis?

b) What is your treatment?

5

Question 5.34

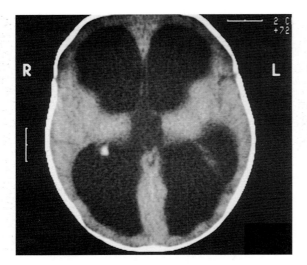

A six-week-old baby was referred with macrocephaly. The baby was born at term after an uneventful pregnancy.

a) What is the diagnosis?

b) List four clinical features.

c) Give two underlying aetiologies.

Question 5.35

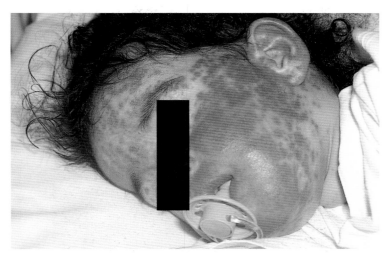

This baby was admitted with a febrile illness. This rash was most pronounced over the face and peripheries where it resembled erythema multiforme. Positive serology for CMV was detected together with mildly abnormal liver function tests.

a) What is the diagnosis?

b) Give two other documented infectious aetiologies.

5

EXAM

QUESTIONS

1

2

3

4

5

6

Case
History Paper

Question 6.1

Jenny, aged 14 years, is referred to the emergency clinic complaining of a loss of sensation and numbness over her left big toe and instep. This sensory loss developed suddenly three weeks after she suffered a minor riding accident when she fell onto a horse jump. Apart from a bruise to her left buttock she is otherwise uninjured. Her general health is good, although she recently had a diarrhoeal illness after a holiday in Greece. Her parents had been similarly unwell with the same illness while on holiday. Jenny was also under the care of the general practitioner three years ago for severe headaches. These responded to simple analgesia. She had had no headaches for one year since, in fact, she had moved schools. She is an only child and her parents are well. The main reason for referral is Jenny's mother's anxiety that this could be the first sign of multiple sclerosis, which had severely debilitated an aunt.

Examination of Jenny's foot confirms a loss of all sensory modalities over the dorsum of her left toe. The rest of her leg is normal and her motor system in both legs is intact. Her tendon reflexes are normal. Examination of her spine is unremarkable. Her buttock is apparently normal, although Jenny felt a diffuse lump over the area where she had fallen at the same time as noticing the loss of sensation. Careful palpation fails to confirm this. Cranial nerve examination and fundoscopy are normal. Bowel and urinary function have not altered. There are no abdominal masses. A soft bruit is heard over her left buttock on careful auscultation. Lower limb pulses and blood pressure measurements are all normal.

The results of investigations performed are as follows:

- Lumbar spine radiograph   Normal
- MRI spine   Normal
- Ultrasound of left buttock   Normal
- Left sural nerve conduction study: Reduced amplitude and velocity of sensory action potential compared to contralateral side.

In view of the lack of improvement in symptoms, Jenny's parents request a lumbar puncture with CSF examination and further CNS imaging:

- CT brain scan   Normal.
- CSF   Normal – no oligoclonal bands detected.

a) What is the likely diagnosis?

b) Give a further diagnostic investigation to confirm the diagnosis.

Question 6.2

A seven-year-old Jamaican boy is admitted to the resuscitation room with a prolonged seizure. He has been unwell for 24 hours with a mild fever and painful throat. His seizure commenced at least 45 minutes before admission. The paramedic team had administered two doses of rectal diazepam 5 mg to no avail. He had suffered a minor head injury 72 hours previously when he fell off a climbing frame. The skull radiograph performed at the time did not reveal a skull fracture. His adoptive mother does not think that he had lost consciousness following the head injury.

On examination, he is convulsing violently in all his limbs. His pupils are dilated and poorly reactive. His plantar reflexes are variable. There is no external evidence of violence. There are no retinal haemorrhages. His Glasgow Coma Score is 5. He responds to a combination of further intravenous diazepam and rectal paraldehyde. Once he stops fitting, further examination reveals small depigmented macules over his right buttock. His fever settles on admission and is 36.7°c on measurement. A systolic murmur is noted and he appears mildly anaemic. Both tympanic membranes are mildly inflamed as are his fauces.

His mother is unable to give a full past medical history as she had only recently adopted him and brought him to the UK. However, while abroad he had received special schooling for behavioural and learning disability. His heart murmur had been clinically diagnosed as a ventriculoseptal defect (VSD).

He undergoes a series of investigations excluding a lumbar puncture, which was deferred in view of the duration of his seizure. The following results are obtained:

- Hb   12.4 g/dl.
- WCC 17.8×10^9/l.
- Platelets 247×10^9/l.
- ESR   12 mm/h.
- Hb electrophoresis Normal pattern.
- CRP   2 mg/l.
- Sodium   128 mmol/l.

- Potassium   3.1 mmol/l.
- Urea   2.1 mmol/l.
- Glucose   11.5 mmol/l.
- Calcium   2.4 mmol/l.
- Phosphate   2.0 mmol/l.
- Magnesium   1.3 mmol/l.
- Chest radiograph   Normal.
- Urinalysis   Negative.
- Blood culture   Negative.
- Urine culture   Negative.
- ECG   Normal.
- Emergency CT brain scan   Periventricular areas that enhance with contrast.

a) What is the most likely diagnosis?

b) What would an echocardiogram reveal?

c) List four other features of this disorder.

Question 6.3

A three-month-old infant is admitted with acute bronchiolitis. She has been ill for four days at home with increasing distress and a deteriorating feeding pattern. Her mother thinks that the infant has become blue on several occasions on the day of admission.

The baby is afebrile on admission and weighs 3.4 kg. Her respiratory rate is 85 per minute and she is grunting. Marked sternal and subcostal recession is noted. Although she is tachycardic, she is not hypotensive and her capillary refill time is two seconds. Her O_2 saturation in air is only 88%, although this improves to 97% in 40% humidified headbox oxygen.

This is the second child born to unrelated parents. She was born at 42 weeks' gestation without major problems, although there had been meconium staining of the liquor at delivery. Her birth weight was 3.15 kg. Breastfeeding was established, but the mother swapped to formula milk after six weeks. There is no significant family history of disease. Both parents are moderate smokers. Mother complains that this baby has always been a 'sicky' baby after feeds, although this had recently improved before this illness. The following results are obtained:

- Hb   12.4 g/dl.
- CRP   3 mg/dl.
- Blood cultures   No growth.
- Electrolytes   All normal.

6

- 24-h oesophageal pH study   Reflux 3%.
- Chest radiograph   First film: hyperexpanded lung fields with suggestion of infiltrates; Second film: right upper lobe collapse.
- Immunofluorescence for RSV/ adenovirus/influenza   Negative.
- Viral culture   Positive for parainfluenza type 3.

Further clinical deterioration necessitated the use of nasal CPAP. General supportive care including intravenous fluids was required. Resolution was slow, with the infant remaining oxygen dependent for three weeks. Eventual improvement was hastened following an empirical trial of inhaled glucocorticosteroids.

a) List three further investigations to elucidate the underlying diagnosis.

b) What is the most likely diagnosis?

c) Outline the further management of this case.

Question 6.4

Simon, a two-year-old boy, is admitted listless and unwell from accident and emergency. He became unwell three days previously. Simon and his two older siblings had returned from a brief holiday in Dorset with their grandparents. During this holiday, Simon and his siblings had suffered gastroenteritis, which granny had blamed upon some poorly cooked beefburgers bought from a promenade kiosk. Simon had been the most unwell with vomiting and diarrhoea. The latter had contained some blood. He had been crying intermittently and pulling his legs up to his chest. However, granny had been able to settle him to sleep. Their food poisoning seemed to settle, so they had returned back home.

On the day of presentation to the hospital, Simon had suffered a brief generalized seizure. His mother was not sure whether he was febrile at the time. He had stopped convulsing by the time his mother had telephoned the general practitioner. He had been seen by his general practitioner who had noted some purpuric spots over his buttocks and elbows and referred him to hospital. He warned Simon's mother that this could be septicaemia or meningitis and had given Simon an injection of parenteral penicillin. When assessed by the paediatric registrar, Simon is pale and tachycardic, but well perfused. He is no more than 2–5% dehydrated and is drinking small volumes regularly. He seems to have recovered from his seizure and although listless, he is alert. His blood pressure is normal for his age. Simon appears a little yellow in the light of the cubicle in accident and emergency. He is therefore admitted for investigation and treatment for possible meningococcaemia.

The results of the investigations are as follows:

- Hb   7.1 g/dl.
- WCC $18 \times 10^9/l$.
- Platelets $45 \times 10^9/l$.
- ESR   45 mm/h.
- Sodium   129 mmol/l.
- Potassium   5.4 mmol/l.
- Urea   25.4 mmol/l.
- Creatinine   146 µmol/l.
- Glucose   12.6 mmol/l.
- Bilirubin   164 µmol/l.
- ALT transaminase   12 IU/l.
- Alkaline phosphatase   98 IU/l.
- Urinalysis   Blood ++, protein ++, specific gravity 1030.

- Blood culture   Sterile.
- Throat swab   Sterile.
- Urine culture   Sterile.
- Urinary antigen for meningococcus   Negative.

a) What is the diagnosis?

b) List two confirmatory investigations.

c) What is the probable culprit accounting for this illness?

d) Outline your subsequent management.

Question 6.5

A three-day-old infant, born at 27 weeks' gestation weighing 731 g, collapses while receiving mechanical ventilation for severe hyaline membrane disease. Initial stabilization following delivery had been accomplished without difficulty. The infant received two doses of exogenous surfactant within the first 18 hours of life with a beneficial response. Ventilatory requirements had remained unchanged for the last 16 hours following transfer to trigger mode ventilation. Current ventilator settings were: peak inspiratory pressure 18 cm H_2O, inspiratory time 0.3 s, FiO_2 0.7. Initial cranial ultrasound scan at four hours of age was normal. The infant is receiving TPN via a percutaneous silastic long line introduced through a left antecubital vein.

Mother is 35 years of age and had a previous preterm infant of 30 weeks' gestation four years ago at another maternity unit. This child had suffered a grade III intraventricular haemorrhage following a pneumothorax associated with severe hyaline membrane disease. In this pregnancy she had received two doses of betamethasone glucocorticosteroid prophylaxis. Mother regularly grew Group B haemolytic streptococci from a vaginal swab during this pregnancy. She had received ampicillin during the delivery of this preterm infant.

The oxygen requirement of this infant had increased for six hours before this collapse. She had become restless. Her sudden oxygen desaturation to 45% prompted reintubation. Thin copious 'secretions' were noted welling out of the trachea, making reintubation difficult. Failure to improve necessitated the use of a cold light source, but no pneumothorax could be demonstrated.

The most recent blood investigation results are:

- Hb   12.9 g/dl.
- Platelets 141×10^9/l.
- WCC 4.6×10^9/l.
- CRP   Less than 1 mg/l.
- Sodium   130 mmol/l.
- Cultures   All no growth.
- pH   7.15.
- P_{CO_2} 8.5 kPa.
- P_{O_2} 3.2 kPa.
- Base excess -3.2.
- Bicarbonate   18 mmol/l.

a) List three potential reasons for the deterioration in this infant's clinical state.

b) List three further investigations to ascertain the cause of the collapse.

c) The chest radiograph reveals a unilateral left side 'white out'. What is the most likely cause?

d) How may this be confirmed?

e) How may this complication be avoided?

Data Interpretation Paper

Question 6.6

A six-year-old boy is referred for assessment before adenotonsillectomy. He has been noted to bruise easily by his mother. The following haematological results are obtained:

- PT   14 s (normal 11.5–14.5).
- Thrombin time   13 s (normal 13–16).
- APTT   58 s (normal 38–51).
- Factor VIIIc   0.31 IU/l (normal 0.5–1.5).
- Factor VIIIRAg   1.6 IU/l (normal 0.5–1.5).
- Ristocetin factor (RiCOF)   0.98 IU/l (normal 0.5–1.5).
- Desmopressin test   Minimal response.

a) What is the diagnosis?

b) What is the desmopressin test?

c) What advice should be given to the ENT team?

Question 6.7

A ten-day-old male infant is admitted with vomiting and systemic collapse. He is noticeably hypotonic and has an icthyotic rash. The following results are obtained:

- Hb   14.2 g/dl.
- Septic screen   No growth.
- Sodium   116 mmol/l.
- Potassium   8.1 mmol/l.
- Urea   11.5 mmol/l.
- Creatinine   51 µmol/l.
- Glucose   2.4 mmol/l.
- 17-hydroxyprogesterone   3 nmol/l (normal 0–10).
- ACTH   89 ng/l (normal 10–50).
- Random cortisol   79 nmol/l (normal 140–690).

a) What is the diagnosis?

b) Give two additional investigations to aid diagnosis.

c) List two other clinical problems associated with the diagnosis.

6

Question 6.8

A 3.7 kg baby born at term is admitted to the neonatal unit at eight hours of age following a generalized seizure. Her mother is attending a drug rehabilitation centre and is apparently stable on daily methadone. The labour was normal and augmentation with syntocinon had not been required. The following results are obtained:

- Septic screen — No growth.
- Sodium — 116 mmol/l.
- Potassium — 3.2 mmol/l.
- Urea — 2.3 mmol/l.
- Glucose — 4.2 mmol/l.
- Plasma osmolality — 253 mOsm/kg.
- Urinary toxicology — Positive for opiates, methadone and cocaine.

a) Give two reasons for the neonatal seizure.

b) Give a pathophysiological mechanism for each of your aetiologies.

Question 6.9

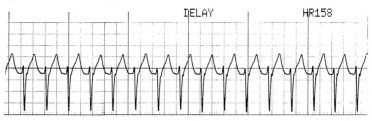

a) What is the interpretation of the investigation?

b) What is your subsequent management?

Question 6.10

A 14-year-old girl is brought to the accident and emergency department with severe facial swelling following a trivial injury. Subsequent investigations reveal:

- Hb   11.4 g/dl.
- IgE   14 IU/l
  (normal concentration 0–40).
- C4   0.1 IU/l
  (normal concentration 0.2–1.7).
- C3   0.4 IU/l
  (normal concentration 0.7–3.4).
- C1q   0.18 g/l (normal concentration).
- C1 inhibitor functional assay   Reduced.

a) What is the diagnosis?

b) What is the appropriate management?

c) What is the mode of inheritance?

Question 6.11

A 15-year-old girl is admitted comatose following a suicide bid. She smells of alcohol and is deeply unconscious. An empty bottle of paracetamol was found in the waste bin at home. Her parents do not know whether this had been discarded previously. Initially she had been hyperventilating when the paramedic team had arrived.

- Arterial pH   7.24.
- P_{O_2} 8.5 kPa.
- P_{CO_2} 3.2 kPa.
- Base excess   −11.
- Bicarbonate   9 mmol.
- Urinalysis   Ketones +++.

a) List four further important investigations.

b) Which other drug is most likely to have been ingested along with the alcohol?

c) Outline your subsequent management.

6

Question 6.12

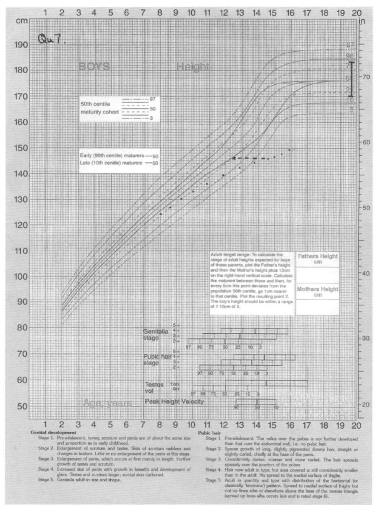

Above is a height chart of a 15-year-old boy.

a) What is the most likely pubertal rating for this boy?

b) What is the most likely diagnosis?

c) List three therapeutic options.

Question 6.13

A six-year-old is admitted with a purpuric rash. The following results are obtained:

- Hb   11.1 g/dl.
- ESR   16 mm/h.
- Platelets $345 \times 10^9/l$.
- PT   14 s.
- APTT   39 s.
- Thrombin time   14 s.
- Antinuclear antibody   Negative.
- Immune complexes   Positive.
- IgG   10 g/l (normal 5–16).
- IgA   3.5 g/l (normal 0.73–2.5).
- IgM   0.9 g/l (normal 0.47–1.7).

a) What is the most likely diagnosis?

b) What is the pathogenesis of the disorder?

c) List three potential complications.

Question 6.14

A 4.9 kg infant aged two days is persistently hypoglycaemic. Current intravenous fluids are 15% dextrose infusion running at 32 ml/h. The following are obtained:

- Glucose   1.8 mmol/l.
- Sodium   133 mmol/l.
- Urea   1.8 mmol/l.
- pH   7.32.
- Cortisol   257 nmol/l.

a) What is the most likely cause of this infant's hypoglycaemia?

b) List two further investigations to aid diagnosis.

c) List three therapeutic options.

6

Question 6.15

A three-year-old boy is admitted for an overnight water deprivation test. His mother claims that he drinks up to four bottles of juice per night and wets the bed at least twice. He also drinks several cups of juice during the day. He is otherwise well and is growing normally. He has recently undergone an adenoidectomy and myringotomies. The results are:

Fast (hours)	Weight (kg)	Urinary osmolality (mOsm/kg)	Plasma osmolality (mOsm/kg)
0	16.4	106	287
6	16.4	456	287
12	16.2	750	290

a) What is the interpretation of the test?

b) What is the cause of his symptoms?

Photographic Material Paper

Question 6.16

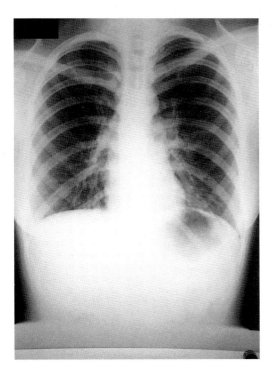

A four-year-old child presented with a persistent cough and fever. Chest examination was largely unremarkable. A blood film identified both haemolysis and rouleaux formation.

a) Describe this chest radiograph.

b) What is the most likely diagnosis?

c) How may this diagnosis be confirmed?

d) List three potential complications.

6

Question 6.17

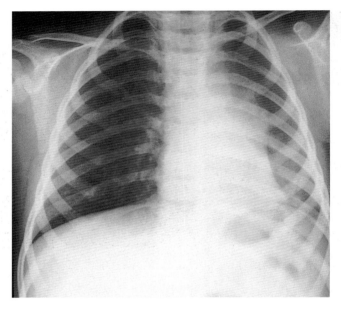

a) What does this chest radiograph show?

b) What is the most likely cause?

c) What is the underlying pathophysiology?

Question 6.18

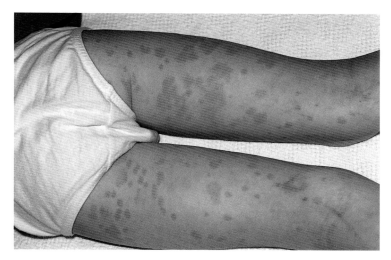

This nine-year-old girl recently suffered a viral-like febrile illness.

a) What is this appearance?

b) List four other potential causes for your diagnosis.

c) What is the treatment?

6

Question 6.19

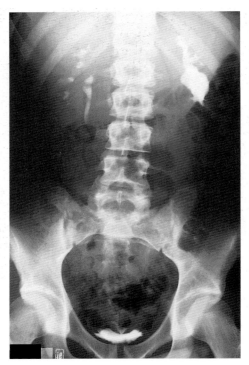

A 15-year-old boy presented with recurrent loin pain. The pain was usually precipitated by illicitly drinking lager.

a) What investigation has been performed?

b) What does it show?

c) What is the link with his intake of alcohol?

Question 6.20

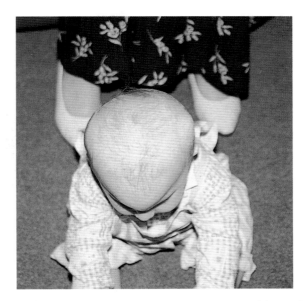

This child was referred because of concerns regarding his head shape.

a) What is the diagnosis?

b) Why has this occurred?

c) What is the treatment?

6

Question 6.21

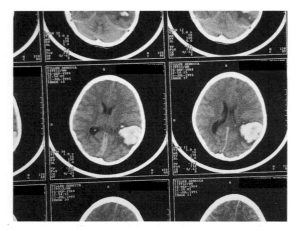

An 11-year-old girl collapsed after a mild viral illness characterized by persistent vomiting. She rapidly became comatose.

a) What is shown?

b) What may be the underlying disorder?

Question 6.22

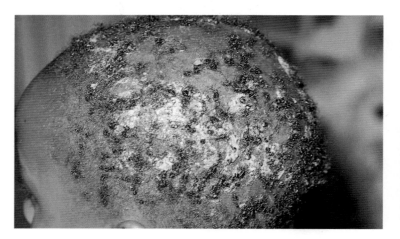

a) What is demonstrated?

b) What is the treatment?

Question 6.23

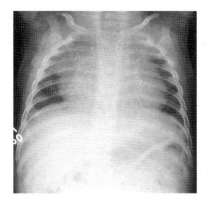

The above chest radiograph was obtained from an infant examined because of a mild upper respiratory tract infection.

a) What is the diagnosis?

b) How may this be proved?

Question 6.24

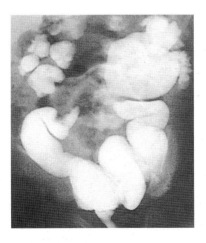

a) What investigation has been performed?

b) What does it demonstrate?

c) Outline your further management.

6

Question 6.25

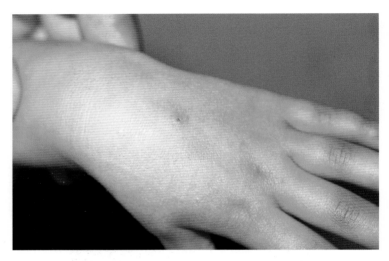

A 12-year-old girl was admitted to the resuscitation room having suffered a generalized seizure. She was unconscious after the seizure was stopped. Her blood glucose was 0.8 mmol/l. Her blood pressure was 80/50 mm Hg. She responded to intravenous dextrose administration.

a) What is demonstrated?

b) What is the likely diagnosis?

c) List four investigations to aid confirmation of the diagnosis.

d) What is your further management?

Question 6.26

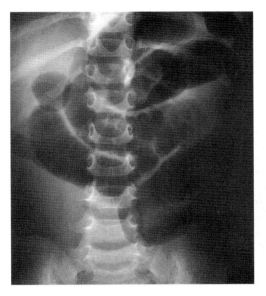

A two-year-old boy is admitted with persistent bilious vomiting.

a) What is the diagnosis?

b) What is your immediate management?

6

Question 6.27

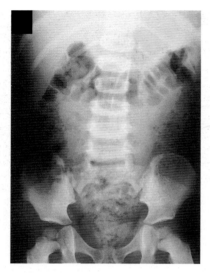

A seven-year-old girl is referred with recurrent abdominal pain.

a) What is the diagnosis?

b) Outline your further management.

Question 6.28

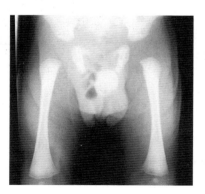

a) What is demonstrated in this radiograph of a preterm infant?

b) Why has this occurred?

Question 6.29

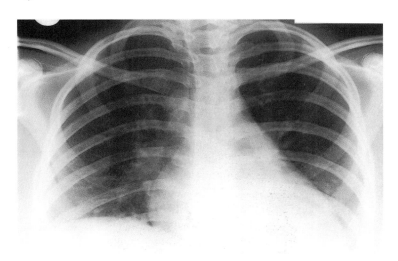

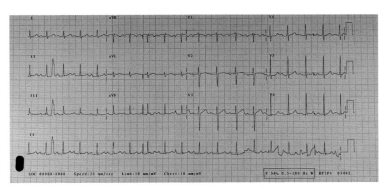

A 14-year-old presented to the accident and emergency department with a swollen knee. Subsequently the patient deteriorated with fever and breathlessness.

a) What does the chest radiograph show?

b) What is the interpretation of the ECG?

c) What is the underlying diagnosis?

d) List four other features of the diagnosis.

e) What is the treatment?

6

Question 6.30

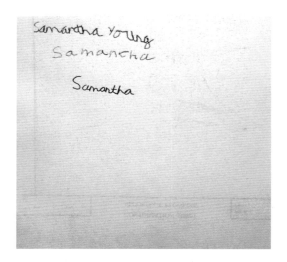

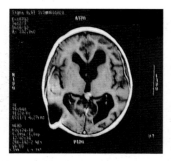

A six-year-old girl underwent neuroimaging. She presented with mild headaches. Her mother had noticed a tremor. Her writing before and after treatment is shown together with her scan.

a) What is the cause of her symptoms?

b) What is the treatment?

c) What is the underlying aetiology?

Question 6.31

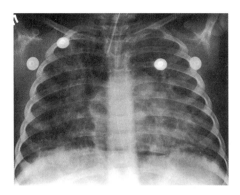

A five-year-old required ventilation after near drowning.

a) What is demonstrated?

b) What is the causative pathophysiology?

c) What are the potential therapeutic interventions available?

Question 6.32

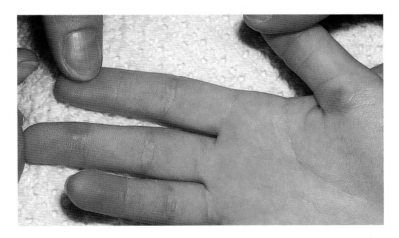

A teenager presented with the above rash on her feet and hands. She also had a sore throat.

a) What is the diagnosis?

b) What is the causative organism?

6

Question 6.33

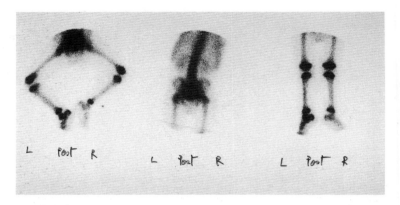

A 23-month-old refuses to weightbear. The ESR and CRP levels are elevated.

a) What investigation has been performed?

b) What is the diagnosis?

c) Outline your treatment.

d) How may the success of your treatment be monitored?

Question 6.34

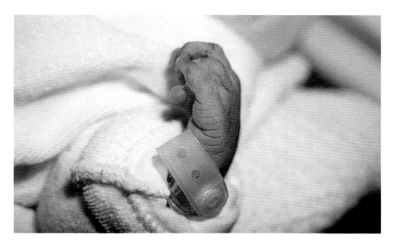

a) What is demonstrated?

b) List four associated disorders.

Question 6.35

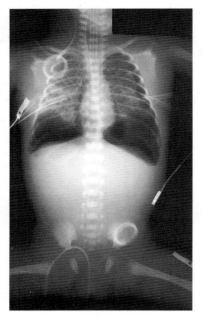

A 25-week-gestation infant was ventilated for prematurity and hyaline membrane disease and suddenly deteriorated.

a) What is the cause of the clinical deterioration?

b) What measures can be adopted to reduce the likelihood of this complication occuring?

EXAM
ANSWERS

1

2

3

4

5

6

ANSWERS – Exam 1

Answer 1.1

a) Chest radiograph: diffuse fine granular shadowing of the lungs. Arterial blood gas: hypoxia; mixed respiratory and metabolic acidosis.

b) Congenital pneumonia with septicaemia.
Obstructed total anomalous pulmonary venous drainage.
Pulmonary haemorrhage.
Aspiration pneumonitis.
Pericardial effusion.
Hypertrophic cardiomyopathy.

Comments   There is evidence of respiratory distress, circulatory failure and hepatomegaly occurring a few hours after birth. One possibility is congenital pneumonia with sepsis, of which Group B streptococcal infection is the commonest cause.

Of the other respiratory causes, the course and gestation are atypical of hyaline membrane disease, and milk aspiration could cause a sudden late respiratory deterioration, but usually without such profound circulatory depression and hepatomegaly. A large pulmonary haemorrhage could cause respiratory distress with this radiological picture and cardiovascular compromise due to acute blood loss, although not hepatomegaly.

Of the cardiac causes, a pericardial effusion is a possibility, but would be expected to cause cardiomegaly and present earlier. Rarely, a hypertrophic cardiomyopathy presents in this way. Total anomalous pulmonary venous drainage is, however, a likelier diagnosis. If the pulmonary veins are obstructed in this condition, it typically presents in the first four days of life with cyanosis and respiratory distress. Pulmonary venous congestion results in the radiological features of pulmonary oedema but there is no cardiomegaly. The obstructed pulmonary veins lead to right-sided cardiac overload and to hepatomegaly. The second heart sound is loud and usually not audibly split. There is poor left-sided cardiac output secondary to reduced left-sided filling. The ECG shows right axis deviation and right ventricular and atrial hypertrophy, but an urgent echocardiogram is required to confirm the diagnosis. This is one of the cardiac lesions that is not picked up on the routine four-chamber view used for antenatal scanning.

Answer 1.2

a) Hyponatraemic dehydration secondary to infectious gastroenteritis (leading to hypovolaemic shock).

b) Correct shock with 10–20 ml/kg boluses of fluid.

c) Cystic fibrosis.

Comments In any case of presumed infectious gastroenteritis where the severity of the dehydration is greater than the history suggests (non-severe diarrhoea and vomiting, fluid tolerance and short duration) an underlying cause must be sought. Further clues here are the pre-existing evidence of failure to thrive despite a good diet and the bronchiolitis illness, whose respiratory symptoms have not settled. Many children with cystic fibrosis have a bronchiolitis-type illness as the initial trigger of their respiratory symptoms. The hyponatraemia and hypokalaemia are secondary to electrolyte losses through skin sweating in a pyrexial child with cystic fibrosis as well as losses in the stool and vomitus, and the blood chloride concentration will also be low. In this case the skin changes, parameters of circulation and tachypnoea are all indicative of shock, which is likely to be hypovolaemic in origin (also suggested by the raised Hb), which must be corrected as the first priority.

Answer 1.3

a) Inhaled foreign body causing right lower lobe pneumonia.
   Persistent mucus plug secondary to viral induced asthma.
   Primary right lower lobe pneumonia.

b) Rigid bronchoscopy with removal of foreign body.

Comments An inhaled foreign body must always be considered in a young mobile child who experiences a sudden onset of respiratory symptoms. In this case there is no initial pyrexia to suggest a primary pneumonia, and although there is mild bronchospasm, this is a common airway response to an inhaled foreign body.

A mucus plug is much less likely to be responsible for the reduced breath sounds of such a mild wheezy episode. The diagnosis of an inhaled foreign body must also be considered in any child with a suspected pneumonia or primary wheezing illness who is not responding to conventional treatment, or indeed, as here, is deteriorating despite therapy. There should be a low threshold for a referral for bronchoscopy in such cases. Rigid bronchoscopy can diagnose and remove the object; fibreoptic bronchoscopy is diagnostic only. A choking episode will have been witnessed in fewer than 50% of cases. A low pitched inspiratory noise or 'thud' may also be heard. In this particular case inhalation of part of a toy while playing was the cause, leading to blockage of the right lower lobe bronchus with subsequent consolidation and atelectasis.

Answer 1.4

a) Right-sided (parietal) skull fracture.
Splaying (widening) of the right coronal suture.

b) Cranial CT or MRI scan.

c) Full skeletal survey.
Neurosurgical opinion.
Ophthalmology review.
Full clotting screen.
Full blood count.
'Child at risk' register check.
Review of previous sibling's death.
Involve local child protection team.
Gather information from all health professionals involved with the care of the baby and both parents.

d) Non-accidental injury causing right-sided skull fracture and underlying subdural haematoma.

Comments Non-accidental injury must always be considered in skeletal injuries where the force is unlikely to have produced the severity of injury, and is even less likely to in young infants who are much less mobile. There are many other clues here, including the delay in seeking help, a child who has been perceived by the parents as having feeding problems and excessive crying (which can lead to parental anxiety and stress) and the previous sibling's death, which is not fully explained. A high index of suspicion needs to be maintained as many cases do not have so many clues at the time of presentation. Whenever a head injury is present (particularly here with the neurological symptoms and tense anterior fontanelle) a cranial CT scan is mandatory, even if the skull radiograph is normal. In this case the skull radiograph was useful, showing a fracture and a localized area of increased pressure (as only the right coronal suture is splayed) under the right parietal region, most likely a bleed, of which the commonest cause in this setting is a subdural haematoma. Some useful information about the presence of previous subdural bleeds, and age of any bleed, may also be obtained from the CT scan.

Neurological stabilization, including a neurosurgical opinion in many cases, is the most important acute step in managing head injury. The further steps listed in c) are essential, and a further interview of the parents will be needed.

In this particular case, a skeletal survey revealed old left-sided multiple rib fractures (posterior and in the mid-axillary line), and ophthalmological examination revealed retinal haemorrhages, which can be seen with intracranial bleeding, not necessarily only in the setting of non-accidental injury. A cranial CT scan confirmed a recent (i.e. later than the rib fractures) right subdural haematoma. The skull fracture and midline shift are also shown.

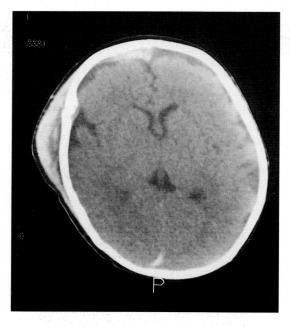

CT scan – right-sided parietal skull fracture with subdural haematoma and blood in the falx.

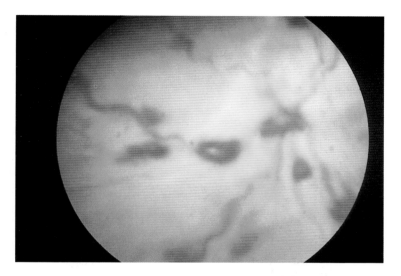

Retinal haemorrhages typical of those found in non-accidental injury.

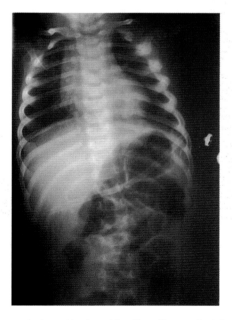

Rib fractures – posteriorly and in the mid axillary line on the left side and probably older than ten days.

Answer 1.5

a) Ensure all the equipment for IPPV and oxygen supply are working and being used correctly.
Check the baby's airway is patent.
Tracheal intubation with IPPV.

b) Left-sided congenital diaphragmatic hernia.
Left-sided tension pneumothorax.
Left pleural effusion.
Right lung collapse.
Right lung hypoplasia.

c) The presence of a scaphoid abdomen points to a diaphragmatic hernia.
Positive chest transillumination points to a pneumothorax.

Comments   The movement of the heart to the right suggests either severe lung atelectasis or hypoplasia on the right side, a mass effect on the left side, or in the absence of respiratory distress, simple dextrocardia. However, the reduced breath sounds on the left suggest a left-sided lung pathology. This suggests a diagnosis of congenital diaphragmatic hernia, pleural effusion or a tension pneumothorax causing mediastinal shift to the right. In the case of congenital diaphragmatic hernia, respiratory distress worsens as gas fills up the bowel in the chest and in exacerbated by bag and mask IPPV. If this diagnosis is suspected, early endotracheal intubation is mandatory, with passage of a nasogastric tube to decompress the bowel.

Spontaneous pneumothoracies are not uncommon, but rarely cause tension pneumothoraces at birth, although co-existent pulmonary hypoplasia may predispose to this complication. If confirmed urgent chest needle thoracocentesis must be carried out followed by a formal chest tube insertion.

A congenital pleural effusion would usually cause respiratory distress from birth, rather than after a few minutes of age, but is still a possible diagnosis.

The basic A(irway) B(reathing) C(irculation) must be followed in neonatal resuscitation, and equipment checked if not producing the desired effect.

Answer 1.6

a) Blood glucose.
   Urinalysis for glycosuria and ketonuria.

b) Diabetes mellitus.

Comments Serum osmolality can be estimated from $2 \times (Na^+ + K^+)$ + glucose + urea. In this case the blood glucose is estimated as 17 mmol/l, but this should be confirmed by biochemical analysis. Assessment for ketoacidosis and dehydration is important in the acute presentation. Diabetes mellitus in childhood may present with acute ketoacidosis, or more insiduously with polyuria, polydipsia, weight loss, abdominal pain and cramps. Infection may precipitate the condition, and should be sought in all cases, but a raised WCC is not always a good guide.

Answer 1.7

a) Obstructive airways disease.

b) Post-bronchodilator spirometry.

Comments The spirometry shows a moderately reduced FEV_1/ FVC ratio, with a preserved FVC, suggestive of an obstructive airways pattern. The PEF is not always very reduced in obstructive airway disease, and more helpful, when available, is the $FEF_{25-75\%}$, which is a more accurate measure of smaller airways obstruction, as seen in asthma. An improvement in spirometry (FEV_1, FEF_{25-75}, PEF) following a bronchodilator challenge indicates reversibility of the obstructive airways disease, and this is most commonly seen in asthma.

Answer 1.8

a) Ventricular septal defect.
   Left ventricular outflow tract obstruction.

Comments An increase in oxygen saturation between the right atrium and right ventricle suggests a left to right shunt at the level of the ventricular septum, and there is an increase in right ventricular pressure as a result. There is a systolic pressure drop of 45 mm Hg between the left ventricle and the ascending aorta, suggesting obstruction of the left ventricular outflow tract. This is most likely to be due to either aortic valve stenosis or subaortic stenosis, and has resulted in a raised left ventricular pressure.

Answer 1.9

a) Methaemoglobinaemia.
   Sulfhaemoglobinaemia.

b) Observation of the blood, which has a chocolate-coloured hue.

c) Methylene blue.
   Vitamin C therapy.

Comments The arterial blood gas shows a high arterial oxygen tension, which excludes a respiratory or cardiac aetiology for the cyanosis in a newborn with a normal Hb level. This leaves methaemoglobinaemia, or less commonly sulfhaemoglobinaemia, as the cause of the cyanosis. 1.5 g/dl of methaemoglobin is sufficient to cause cyanosis, but the oxygen-carrying capacity of the blood is not usually affected until about 30–50% of the Hb is in the methaemoglobin form. The iron in the ferric (nonfunctional) form imparts a chocolate hue to the blood. Since the introduction of nitric oxide therapy, many hospitals have access to rapid methaemoglobin level analysis. The most commonly used reducing agents (converting the haem iron back from the ferric to the normal ferrous state) are methylene blue and vitamin C, and these are therapeutic in most causes of methaemoglobinaemia. The reason for the low oxygen saturation on pulse oximetry in this condition is the different spectral absorption of methaemoglobin in comparison with oxyhaemoglobin, which makes pulse oximetry inaccurate.

Answer 1.10

a) Electromechanical dissociation.

b) Secure the airway.
   Ventilate with high concentration of oxygen.
   Adrenaline 10 µg/kg intravenously or intraosseously.
   Volume replacement (typically 20 ml/kg) intravenously or intra-osseously.

c) Hypovolaemia from acute blood loss.
   Tension pneumothorax from chest trauma.
   Cardiac tamponade.
   Pulmonary embolus.
   Hypothermia.

Comments Electromechanical dissociation is the absence of any palpable pulses despite the presence of recognizable complexes on the

ECG monitor. The commonest cause in childhood is severe shock making it difficult to feel the pulses. The causes listed above must be sought and actively treated. Possible causes in other situations include drug overdose and electrolyte imbalance.

Answer 1.11

a) Hypochromia.
Microcytosis.

b) α-thalassaemia trait.

c) None.

Comments The blood results show microcytic hypochromic erythrocytes, but no anaemia. The normal ferritin excludes iron deficiency as the cause providing there is no co-existing inflammatory process. In β-thalassaemia there is usually a raised HbA_2, and microcytosis is more marked. α-thalassaemia trait is most often seen in children from the Mediterranean and South East Asia, and is uncommon among Western European populations. Definitive diagnosis requires measuring globin chain synthesis, which is not currently in routine clinical use. Anaemia is seen in only a proportion of patients. In lead poisoning the red cells show basophilic stippling; a raised erythrocyte zinc protoporphyrin may help in the diagnosis. Serum iron concentration is typically raised in sideroblastic anaemia.

Answer 1.12

a) Allergic bronchopulmonary aspergillosis (ABPA).

b) Fleeting fluffy patchy changes.

c) Oral glucocorticosteroids.

Comments ABPA must be considered in any child with cystic fibrosis who has either a predominantly wheezing illness, or a suspected infective exacerbation that fails to respond to appropriate antibiotics. A dramatic increase in total IgE concentration is seen, and as most children with cystic fibrosis have an IgE measurement as part of their annual assessment bloods, an acute rise from baseline, as here, may be seen. Specific IgE to *Aspergillus fumigatus*, *Aspergillus precipitins* and immediate skin sensitivity may provide supporting evidence, but *Aspergillus* is only occasionally cultured from the sputum. A chest radiograph may give valuable information. In this case the clinical features with the raised total IgE concentration and negative sputum culture make

ABPA more likely than an infective or bronchoconstrictive exacerbation of cystic fibrosis. Systemic antifungals are of no value in treatment, which should be with oral glucocorticosteroids, often a long course (several months). ABPA may occur in other chronic pulmonary conditions including asthma.

Answer 1.13

a) A low CD4+ T lymphocyte concentration and hypergammaglobulinaemia.

b) Anti-HIV IgG antibody testing after counselling.

Comments   The results show a low CD4+ T lymphocyte count, both in absolute terms (a concentration of $0.4 \times 10^9/l$ or less is abnormal at any age) and as a percentage of the total lymphocyte count (a concentration less than 15% at any age indicates severe immunosuppression from HIV infection). Nonetheless, it must be remembered that normal CD4+ counts are higher in early childhood, and children can develop opportunistic infections at higher CD4+ concentration than adults. Chronic diarrhoea can be caused by HIV infection, but bacterial, mycobacterial, parasitic and fungal infections may involve the gastrointestinal tract in HIV infection.

Answer 1.14

a) Hypsarrhythmia.

b) Infantile spasms.

Comments   The EEG shows typical features of hypsarrhythmia, with a chaotic background of high amplitude slow activity and multifocal spikes over both hemispheres. Hypsarrhythmia is sometimes unilateral or asymmetrical, or may appear only during sleep. It is typically associated with infantile spasms, a form of generalized myoclonic seizures occurring during infancy. These seizures represent a nonspecific reaction of immature cerebral cortex to injury or abnormal growth and development, most commonly cerebral (especially perinatal) anoxia or cerebral malformations, as occur in tuberous sclerosis and Down syndrome.

Answer 1.15

a) Obstruction to urine excretion from the left kidney, not relieved by frusemide.

b) Pelvi-ureteric junction obstruction.
Vesico-ureteric junction obstruction.
Other lesions within the ureter (e.g. calculus) or compressing from
the outside (e.g. tumour, lymph node).

Comments A normal renogram shows a peak of uptake at around
4–5 minutes, followed by a steady decline, representing excretion of the
contrast. This is the case here for the right kidney, but the left kidney
shows continuing uptake, representing a failure of renal excretion. A
response to frusemide usually indicates a functional obstruction, but
here there is a failure to respond to frusemide. This indicates an organic
obstruction, most often at the pelvi-ureteric junction, but sometimes at
the vesico-ureteric junction.

Answer 1.16

a) Horizontal earlobe crease.
Associated with Beckwith (–Wiedemann) syndrome.

b) Hypoglycaemia.

Comments Hypoglycaemia is a common feature of Beckwith
(–Wiedemann) syndrome in the neonatal period. It is due to hyperinsulinism and is often prolonged and severe. Macrosomia, macroglossia,
exomphalos, hemihypertrophy, visceromegaly (especially of the liver)
and renal medullary dysplasia may all be present. Polycythaemia, facial
naevus and mild microcephaly are also features.

Answer 1.17

a) Bilateral Harrison's sulci.

b) Poorly controlled asthma.

Comments Harrison's sulci (or grooves) are seen at the costal inser-
tions of the diaphragm. They are seen in any condition with increased
activity of the diaphragm. This is most commonly due to respiratory
conditions with increased work of breathing, including poorly controlled chronic asthma, upper airways obstruction and cardiac conditions with significant left to right shunts. They may be present in severe
rickets due to a poorly compliant thoracic cage.

Answer 1.18

a) Air in the right pleural cavity.
Fluid in the right pleural cavity.
Incomplete collapse of the right lung.

b) Right-sided pyopneumothorax or empyema with bronchopleural fistula.
Pleural effusion with attempted drainage allowing air to enter from outside.

Comments   This appearance is most commonly seen with a pyopneumothorax, most commonly arising from underlying lung infection. The infection spreads to the pleural space, and particularly in severe or prolonged infections, as here, an airleak (bronchopleural fistula) may develop, hence the appearance of air in the pleural space. In thoracic empyema, a thick fibrinous rind forms around the lung, limiting its re-expansion. Another possible explanation for the appearances is insertion of an intercostal chest drain (not present here) or a needle thoracocentesis for pleural fluid drainage, allowing air to enter from the outside. A traumatic hydropneumothorax is unlikely as there is no evidence of a rib fracture and the incomplete right lung collapse suggests a lung pathology.

Answer 1.19

a) Henoch–Schönlein vasculitis/purpura.

b) Throat swab for culture.
Urinalysis for protein and blood.
Urine microscopy for red cells and casts.
Elevated antibody titre to streptococcal antigen (anti-streptolysin O titre, anti-DNase B).

Comments   The cause of Henoch–Schönlein vasculitis is unknown, but it may follow an upper respiratory infection, occasionally streptococcal in origin. The typical rash is not always the first manifestation of the disease, and is often urticarial or maculopapular in nature at first, but then becomes purpuric or petechial. The rash may then suggest a bleeding diathesis or septicaemia, and these must be excluded. The rash distribution is usually over the buttocks and extensor surfaces of the legs, and occasionally the arms, as well as the trunk and face. Other rashes may be present, including erythema multiforme, and angioedema may occur. Gastrointestinal complications, arthritis and neurological manifestations may all occur in the acute phase. Renal involvement is potentially the most serious manifestation, occurring in 25–50% of children in the acute phase, with 3–5% progressing to chronic renal failure.

Answer 1.20

a) Child sexual abuse.
Lichen sclerosis et atrophicus.
Vulvovaginitis.
Threadworm or pinworm infection.
Streptococcal infection.

Comments This child had histologically confirmed lichen sclerosis et atrophicus, a skin condition of uncertain aetiology that is often itchy. The lesions are typically shiny and ivory-coloured, with violaceous margins. The anogenital region, as here, is commonly affected, but other parts may also be involved. Child sexual abuse must be excluded when this appearance is seen, and when only the genital region is involved. Chronic primary vulvovaginitis gives a similar appearance. Threadworm, pinworm or streptococcal infection may cause anogenital inflammation from itching and scratching, but not such atrophic shiny skin.

Answer 1.21

a) Frayed metaphyses.
Widened (splayed) metaphyses.
Cupped metaphyses.
Osteopaenia of the shafts and epiphyses.

b) Active rickets.

c) Reduced growth.
Craniotabes with widely patent or delayed closure of anterior fontanelle.
Rachitic rosary.
Swollen wrists and ankles.
Bow legs (commoner once weight-bearing).

Comments Rickets may arise from a number of causes of which nutritional deficiency of vitamin D is the most common. Others include conditions in which there is interference with metabolic conversion and activation of vitamin D, such as renal and hepatic lesions, or with calcium and phosphorus homeostasis. The radiological appearance shown here is characteristic, and treatment depends upon the cause.

Answer 1.22

a) Anogenital warts.

b) Sexual abuse.

Comments   Anogenital warts are caused by human papilloma virus (HPV) infection. In all cases of anogenital warts, a careful history and examination must be carried out to exclude the possibility of child sexual abuse, although most infections are transmitted non-sexually. The presence of similar lesions in other family members does not necessarily imply sexual transmission, as spread by innocent hand touching is common. Typing using DNA probes is not valuable as both genital and extragenital HPV types may be found in these lesions.

Answer 1.23

a) Right-sided pulmonary embolism secondary to infective endocarditis. Right-sided segmental pneumonia.

b) Ventilation–perfusion scan, which will show normal ventilation with absent perfusion to the affected area.
Pulmonary angiography (more invasive), which will show the embolus.

Comments   Left to right shunts (as here with a ventricular septal defect) result in right-sided vegetations (typically at the site where the jet of blood through the defect impinges on the ventricular wall) when infective endocarditis occurs. Embolism of the vegetation is therefore likely to be to the lungs, resulting in respiratory distress, hypoxia, chest pain and cough, and occasionally haemoptysis. Chest radiography may, as here, show a classical wedge-shaped infarct (the lower lobes are most commonly affected), and this is best confirmed by a ventilation–perfusion scan. Pulmonary angiography will show the site of embolism and may be used therapeutically for embolectomy. Echocardiography and serial blood cultures must be carried out, and aggressive antibiotic therapy started.

Answer 1.24

a) Miliary tuberculosis.

b) Culture of CSF (contraindicated if there is evidence of raised intracranial pressure).
Serial early morning urines and gastric aspirates.
Tuberculin skin test.
Bronchoscopy with lavage and transbronchial lung biopsy.

Comments Miliary tuberculosis results from haematogenous spread of *Mycobacterium tuberculosis*, and in children is most commonly seen in infants. It is rare in developed countries, but with the increased incidence of AIDS, the incidence may rise. BCG is protective, but tuberculin skin testing is often negative, probably due to overwhelming disease. A chest radiograph showing bilateral miliary infiltrates, as here, is diagnostic, but in other cases CSF, lung, gastric and urine cultures may be necessary.

Answer 1.25

a) Cardiomegaly.
   Bilateral perihilar shadowing consistent with pulmonary venous congestion.

b) Viral myocarditis.
   Viral pericarditis.
   Pericardial effusion.

Comments The onset of cardiac failure following a history of an upper respiratory and gastrointestinal infection suggests a myocarditis, most likely viral in aetiology. Myocarditis usually presents with symptoms and signs of cardiac failure, and occasionally with arrhythmias, and there may be evidence of a preceding infectious illness. Diagnosis is best made by echocardiography, which typically demonstrates global cardiac enlargement with atrioventricular valve regurgitation and poorly contracting ventricles. Various viral, bacterial, fungal, protozoal, rickettsial and spirochaetal infections may cause infectious myocarditis, the commonest being the enteroviruses, particularly coxsackie B and echovirus. Other causes of cardiomyopathy must be borne in mind.

Answer 1.26

a) Gas in the bowel wall (pneumatosis intestinalis).

b) Necrotizing enterocolitis.

Comments Necrotizing enterocolitis must be considered in any preterm neonate with gastrointestinal symptoms and signs, unexplained acute deterioration, or suspected sepsis. Abdominal radiography may show gas in the bowel wall, which is diagnostic, but early on may be normal or reveal only mild nonspecific bowel dilatation in the condition. Portal vein gas is seen later, and pneumoperitoneum indicates a perforation.

Answer 1.27

a) Imperforate anus.
   Rectovaginal fistula.

Comments It is important to distinguish between a 'high' and 'low' anomaly when anorectal atresia is found. The presence of an external fistula to the perineum or vestibule (as here) indicates a 'low' lesion. Associated anomalies, particularly of the VATER (vertebral, anorectal, tracheo-oesophageal, renal/radial) association, must be sought.

Answer 1.28

a) Collodion baby.

b) Cutaneous infection.
   Dehydration.
   Respiratory distress.

Comments The collodion baby is covered at birth by a thick shiny membrane, which can restrict underlying tissues. The condition is typically a manifestation of ichthyosis. Shedding usually starts soon after birth, and can be hastened by maintenance in a high humidity environment. A careful watch for cutaneous infection and dehydration with electrolyte imbalance must be maintained.

Answer 1.29

a) Intussusception (an echodense lesion, the apex of the intussusception, surrounded by an echolucent area, which is the gas within the bowel into which the intussusception is occurring, the intussuscipiens).

Comments In doubtful clinical cases of intussusception, ultrasound is now commonly used to assist in aiding diagnosis. In some centres, air or barium reduction of the intussusception is performed under ultrasound control, although in most centres fluoroscopic guidance is used. This procedure is contraindicated in the presence of peritonism or bowel obstruction, in which case urgent surgery is necessary.

Answer 1.30

a) Left upper lobe congenital lobar emphysema.
   Left-sided congenital lung cyst.
   Cystic adenomatoid malformation.

Comments Left upper lobe congenital lobal emphysema is caused by a congenital ball valve effect of the affected lobar bronchus, occasionally secondary to extrinsic compression. Presentation is usually within the first few weeks of life with respiratory distress and reduced breath sounds over the affected area. Chest radiography within the first 24–48 hours may be normal as lung fluid is clearing. The left upper lobe is most commonly affected, and diagnosis should be confirmed using a ventilation–perfusion lung scan and a CT scan, as simple chest radiography may give similar appearances to congenital lung cysts, particularly a type III congenital cystic adenomatoid malformation of the lung. Those with absent ventilation and perfusion on lung scan or symptoms need surgical resection of the affected lobe.

Answer 1.31

a) Hypertrophy or pseudohypertrophy of the calves.

b) Duchenne muscular dystrophy (DMD).

c) Creatine kinase.
DNA analysis.
Muscle biopsy.
Electromyography.

Comments The usual presentation of a boy with DMD is with an apparent deterioration in motor skills or delayed onset of walking beyond the usual upper limit of 18 months. Global developmental delay is a common feature. Typical clinical features are tight Achilles' tendons and (shown here) prominent calves, caused by fatty replacement of normal muscle. The DMD gene has been cloned and this codes for a cell membrane protein called dystrophin. With current laboratory techniques about 65% of the deletions of this gene can be detected, so more invasive diagnostic techniques such as muscle biopsy and electromyography can be reserved for those cases in whom DNA analysis is normal.

Answer 1.32

a) Finger bruising.

Comments A full clinical evaluation is warranted in this situation to establish the exact mechanism of injury. A diagnosis of non-accidental injury should be considered for all unusual skin lesions and all injuries that are not consistent with the given mechanism of injury or out of keeping with the age of the child. Thorough notekeeping with illustrations is essential; radiology may be indicated for evidence of healed fractures (either radiographs or, in older children, a bone scan), and clotting and platelet studies are often needed for bruising.

Answer 1.33

a) A micturating cystourethrogram.

b) Dilated posterior urethra.
   Transverse linear filling defect proximal to dilated urethra.
   Bladder diverticula.
   Thickened bladder wall.
   Diagnosis: posterior urethral valves.

Comments Posterior urethral valves must be suspected in any infant boy presenting with urinary tract infection, poor urinary stream or impaired renal function. Most cases are now diagnosed at birth as a result of antenatal ultrasound screening showing hydronephrotic kidneys and distended bladder. If the diagnosis is strongly suspected, a micturating cystourethrogram should be performed. Most (though not all!) urologists and paediatricians would agree that this should be performed using a suprapubic catheter, as urethral catheterization may partially disrupt the valves, making surgery more difficult.

Answer 1.34

a) Midline space-occupying lesion in the posterior fossa.
   Low attenuation signals surrounding the lesion (due to oedema).
   Obliteration of the fourth ventricle.

Comments Of the neoplasms found in the posterior fossa, cerebellar astrocytoma, medulloblastoma and ependymoma are the commonest. Presenting symptoms may be related to raised intracranial pressure, such as headache, early morning vomiting and sixth nerve palsy, cerebellar signs, or other more vague symptoms such as change in behaviour, particularly irritability. MRI is more sensitive, and should be performed if the CT scan is negative and the diagnosis is still in doubt.

Answer 1.35

a) Right Erb (–Duchenne) palsy.

b) Maternal diabetes mellitus.

Comments   In Erb's (or Erb–Duchenne) palsy, there is damage to the fifth and sixth cervical nerves of the brachial plexus. This results in the typical adducted and internally rotated arm, with pronation of the forearm. Differentiation must be made from cerebral injury and damage to the clavicle or humerus. It most commonly occurs when there is difficulty in delivering the baby's shoulders, which most commonly happens in babies with macrosomia, as is the case with many infants of mothers with diabetes mellitus.

EXAM
ANSWERS

1
2
3
4
5
6

ANSWERS – Exam 2
Answer 2.1

a) Pauciarticular juvenile chronic arthritis (JCA).

b) Antinuclear antibody (ANA) titre.
   Ophthalmological assessment for iridocyclitis.

c) Nephritis secondary to use of non-steroidal anti-inflammatory drugs.
   Renal amyloid.

2

Comments There is evidence of inflammation of the joints, supported by mildly raised inflammatory parameters in the blood. An
infectious cause is unlikely given the lack of pyrexia or systemic upset,
the joints involved and the duration of symptoms. The joints involved
are atypical for tuberculosis, which most commonly affects the hip joint
and spine. JCA is often diagnosed after excluding blood dyscrasias, neo-
plastic disorders and collagen or vascular disorders. The duration of the
history in an otherwise well child of this age with no other symptoms or
signs makes these other diagnoses unlikely, but further tests may be
needed to completely exclude them. In pauciarticular JCA in females,
the age of onset is usually less than 5 years of age, and the knee, ankle,
wrist and hand are the most commonly involved joints. Iridocyclitis
must be screened for regularly, and its presence correlates with ANA
positivity. Although amyloid is more common in systemic onset JCA, it
can be seen in all forms of JCA, but more often occurs after a longer
period of unremitting disease than here.

Answer 2.2

a) Erb (Erb–Duchenne) palsy of the left arm.
   Fracture of the left clavicle.
   Fracture or dislocation of the humerus (less commonly).

b) Elevation of the left hemidiaphragm (due to left phrenic nerve palsy).
   Left lung pneumothorax/atelectasis/pleural effusion.
   Diaphragmatic hernia.
   Transient tachypnoea of the newborn.
   Hyaline membrane disease.
   Congenital pneumonia.

c) Fluoroscopic screening of the diaphragm.
   Ultrasound screening of the diaphragm.

Comments Difficulty in delivering the shoulders, a condition called
'shoulder dystocia' is seen with macrosomic babies, the commonest

cause of which is an infant of a diabetic mother. Lateral traction on the head and neck or excessive traction on the shoulders may injure the upper C5 and C6 nerves of the brachial plexus leading to an Erb (Erb–Duchenne) palsy or a skeletal fracture, typically of the clavicle. Less commonly a fracture or dislocation of the humerus or epiphyseal separation may be seen. When the C4 nerve is also affected, phrenic nerve injury is a potential problem and causes respiratory distress as a result of diaphragmatic paralysis on the affected side. Chest radiography in this case may suggest the diagnosis if the left hemidiaphragm is one intercostal space higher than the right (with a right-sided palsy the right hemidiaphragm is usually two intercostal spaces higher than the left). Fluoroscopic screening of the diaphragm is the most commonly used technique to confirm the diagnosis, looking for elevation of the diaphragm on the affected side, and seesaw movements of the diaphragm during respiration. Ultrasound is used more commonly now to make a diagnosis, and phrenic nerve conduction studies are available in some centres.

A spontaneous pneumothorax is a possibility, but other lung conditions predisposed to by the maternal diabetes mellitus, such as transient tachypnoea of the newborn and hyaline membrane disease, are unlikely in view of the clinical data given.

Answer 2.3

a) Typhoid fever or paratyphoid fever (enteric fever).
   Other tropical infections (e.g. inadequately treated malaria).
   Brucellosis.
   Tuberculosis.
   Other bacterial septicaemias including bacterial endocarditis.
   Viral illnesses including hepatitis A.
   Cytomegalovirus (CMV) infection.
   Infectious mononucleosis.
   HIV.

b) Haemolytic anaemia.

c) Glucose-6-phosphate dehydrogenase (G6PD) deficiency.

Comments Typhoid and paratyphoid present in a similar manner, although typhoid is frequently a more severe illness. The incubation period for typhoid fever varies from 1–3 weeks in most cases. The fever then gradually increases and when established there is often a relative bradycardia, though this feature is less common in young children. There may be diarrhoea (particularly in the young child) or constipation, and an interstitial pneumonitis may occur. During the second week there is frequently a major change in the mental state. Rose spots are seen from day seven, characteristically over the trunk, but are only visible in fair-skinned patients. Proteinuria is a frequent finding in typhoid fever, as in many other acute febrile illnesses, and is nonspecific. The WCC is often normal or low, and there may be a relative lymphocytosis.

The absence of diarrhoea and lymphadenopathy rules out a number of possible differential diagnoses, but excluding malaria requires repeated thick and thin blood smears. Other non-infectious diagnoses (e.g. vasculitis, malignancy) must always be borne in mind despite the history of foreign travel, but are unlikely in this case. A haemolytic anaemia may occur due to typhoid itself in G6PD deficient patients, but an alternative mechanism in this patient is drug-induced, from the chloroquine given to treat the clinical diagnosis of malaria. Chloroquine does not precipitate haemolysis as commonly as other antimalarials in G6PD deficiency. A diagnosis of G6PD deficiency in this case is also suggested by the neonatal jaundice, which frequently occurs on day 2–3 of life.

Answer 2.4

a) Partially compensated metabolic acidosis.

b) Cardiovascular status (blood pressure, pulse, capillary refill time).
Blood glucose estimation.
FBC–PCV.

c) Absence of the ventricular system (lateral ventricles).
Poor differentiation of the sulci.
Poor grey/white matter differentiation.

d) Blood glucose concentration.
Blood calcium concentration.
Acid–base balance.
Serum electrolytes.

e) Hypoxic–ischaemic encephalopathy (HIE).
Sepsis with meningo-encephalitis.
Inborn error of metabolism.
Drug withdrawal.

Comments HIE is the commonest neurological problem affecting term neonates. There may be clues such as poor fetal growth in more longstanding cases, meconium staining of the liquor (as here), abnormal fetal heart trace on the cardiotocograph and low fetal scalp or cord pH. However, none of these are diagnostic, and in some cases there may be no clues until the birth. Initial resuscitation consists of achieving adequate oxygenation and adequate cardiovascular status, frequently consisting of volume resuscitation, and then in many cases use of inotropes. Correction of acccompanying metabolic acidosis frequently occurs spontaneously, but judicious partial correction with bicarbonate may be indicated if the pH remains less than 7.1. Babies born with HIE may have hypoglycaemia, which is often present at birth, and hypocalcaemia may occur. If renal function is compromised persistent metabolic acidosis and hyperkalaemia may occur, and at all times physiological homeostasis (e.g. temperature) and biochemical (including acid–base) stability must be maintained as far as possible. Although a cranial CT scan is shown here, in most cases adequate cranial information can be obtained from a cranial ultrasound scan looking for 'slit-like' or obliterated ventricles and diffuse bright echos in the cerebral cortex, suggesting cerebral oedema. Ultrasound scanning is much more easily obtained, and does not require moving a sick baby. Mannitol, restriction of fluids, steroids, judicious hyperventilation and hypothermia have all been used in an attempt to reduce cerebral oedema with variable success, and several neuroprotective agents are currently under investigation. The timing of the hypoxic–ischaemic insult can often be very difficult. In this case, the relatively early onset of fits and meconium staining of the liquor at rupture of the membranes suggest that the insult may have been before the onset of labour or in its early stages.

In all cases good notekeeping is essential for clinical purposes, but this is especially important in cases of suspected HIE, which is a frequent cause of medical litigation, often occurring many years after the event when the surviving child has more needs.

Sepsis with coexistent meningo-encephalitis must always be excluded by appropriate cultures, although lumbar puncture may have to be deferred due to the instability of the baby. Appropriate antibiotics should be commenced until sepsis is excluded. As only 10% dextrose has been given, an inborn error of metabolism is unlikely. Drug withdrawal, most commonly from maternal opiate abuse, is unlikely to cause raised intracranial pressure and the CT scan features described.

Answer 2.5

a) Toxic shock syndrome (TSS).
   Kawasaki disease.
   Drug-induced (penicillin).
   Acute bacterial infections including streptococcal infection and endocarditis.

Viral infections causing hepatitis including infectious mononucleosis.
Tuberculosis.
Malignancy (e.g. leukaemia).
Vasculitis.
Juvenile chronic arthritis.

b) Echocardiogram.
Creatine kinase (CK).
Isolation of staphylococcal toxins.
Presence of antineutrophil cytosolic antibodies (ANCA) and anti-endothelial cell antibodies (AECA).
Viral serology and isolation.
Monospot.
Bone marrow examination.
Chest radiograph.
Tuberculin skin testing.
Blood cultures.
Streptococcal antigen detection.
Other autoantibodies (e.g. anti-dsDNA).

Comments There is a potentially large differential diagnosis for a pyrexial child including a number of infections, malignancies and drug-induced and other chronic inflammatory processes including vasculitis, juvenile chronic arthritis and inflammatory bowel disease. The main features in this case are fever, conjunctivitis, mucous membrane changes, rash, lymphadenopathy, hepatitis and cardiovascular compromise for over five days. This constellation points strongly to either TSS or Kawasaki disease. It is becoming increasingly apparent that there is considerable overlap between these two conditions. Although Kawasaki disease is also called mucocutaneous lymph node syndrome, several cases have no significant lymphadenopathy. It is most common in children under five years of age. Although gastrointestinal upset and particularly generalized myalgia are more often seen in TSS, they may be present in Kawasaki disease. Hepatomegaly and abnormal liver function tests may be seen in both conditions, and in Kawasaki disease there may be hydrops of the gall bladder. The urinary findings are nonspecific and can occur in these and many other febrile conditions. In both TSS and Kawasaki disease there can be cardiovascular compromise: in the latter there may be myocarditis, myocardial ischaemia or infarction, pericarditis and mitral regurgitation, whereas in TSS there is septic shock often with myocardial depression. The platelet count in Kawasaki disease in the first week is often normal, rising subsequently. Echocardiography showing coronary artery dilatation or aneurysm suggests a diagnosis of Kawasaki disease; a low platelet count as here (occasionally with evidence of DIC) and a raised CK point towards a diagnosis of TSS. ANCA and AECA are present in some cases of Kawasaki disease and may therefore be helpful in the differential diagnosis.

Answer 2.6

a) Chronic renal failure.
   Renal osteodystrophy or rickets.
   Acute renal failure.

b) Neuropathic bladder.

c) Establish bladder drainage with urethral catheter.
   Antibiotic treatment for urinary tract infection.
   Treatment of renal osteodystrophy.

Comments Chronic renal failure is an inevitable consequence of neuropathic bladder associated with spina bifida when adequate bladder drainage has not been established. Radiological and urodynamic investigations will determine the best form of long-term bladder drainage. These include intermittent urethral catheterization, indwelling urethral catheter and bladder augmentation, depending upon the type of neuropathic bladder and the patient's motivation and understanding. Successful bladder drainage and treatment of the urinary tract infection in this case should improve the renal function. Hypertension must be actively sought and treated. Other measures, including treatment of the renal osteodystrophy (as here), appropriate diet and treatment of significant acidosis are secondary measures.

Answer 2.7

a) Proximal renal tubular acidosis (RTA).

b) Phosphaturia.
   Glycosuria.
   Aminoaciduria.

Comments Proximal RTA results from reduced proximal tubular reabsorption of bicarbonate. As distal tubular bicarbonate reabsorption remains intact the urine can be acidified, in contrast to distal RTA where urinary pH is always greater than 5.8. Loss of sodium bicarbonate results in hyperchloraemia and hypokalaemia. Proximal RTA may occur as an isolated sporadic or hereditary disorder, or when there is associated phosphaturia, glycosuria and aminoaciduria (frequently leading to polyuria and polydipsia) as part of Fanconi's syndrome. In the case of the latter a search for underlying causes should be made, the commonest of these being cystinosis.

Answer 2.8

a) Diabetes insipidus.

b) Vasopressin (desmopressin or DDAVP™) challenge.

Comments Failure to concentrate urine in diabetes insipidus results in a predisposition to episodes of severe dehydration, often beginning in infancy in the more severe forms of this condition. A water deprivation test should be performed only after other simpler tests, and only by experienced practitioners with adequate supervision. Despite fasting for only four hours there has been a nearly 5% drop in body weight, at which time the test is appropriately ended. At the end of the 4-hour fast there is a raised serum osmolality of 305 mOsm/kg $(2 \times (Na + K)$ + urea + glucose) and an inappropriately dilute urine which confirm the diagnosis. To distinguish between nephrogenic and central diabetes insipidus, an intranasal or intramuscular dose of vasopressin (desmopressin) is given and urine and serum osmolality are measured before, and hourly for four hours after its administration. If the urinary serum osmolality ratio remains less than 1.0, then the diagnosis is of nephrogenic rather than central diabetes insipidus.

2

Answer 2.9

a) Short P–R interval.
   Delta wave.
   Widened QRS complex.

b) Wolff–Parkinson–White (WPW) syndrome.

Comments In WPW syndrome there is an accessory atrioventricular (AV) pathway bypassing the AV node. When this pathway is in use the characteristic ECG pattern shown here is present. This predisposes to supraventricular tachycardia, at which time the ECG features disappear. It is most commonly present in a normal heart, but occasionally it is associated with Ebstein's anomaly, corrected transposition, atrial septal defect and cardiomyopathy. For this age (nine months) the normal range for P–R interval is 0.09–0.13 s and for QRS duration 0.04–0.08 s.

Answer 2.10

a) Swallowed maternal blood from maternal cracked nipples.

Comments Rectal bleeding is not an uncommon problem. Bleeding from the baby's gastrointestinal tract may be due to vitamin K deficiency, thrombocytopaenia, necrotizing enterocolitis, a localized gastrointestinal lesion (e.g. polyp or Meckel's diverticulum) and occasionally milk intolerance. All these must be considered. An alternative common cause is swallowed maternal blood, either during delivery or from cracked nipples in breastfed babies. Typically the bleeding occurs on day 2–4; there may also be vomit containing blood. Differentiation from bleeding from the baby's gastrointestinal tract is based on the presence of fetal haemoglobin in the baby which resists alkali. This forms the basis of the Apt test, where a yellow–brown colour change takes place when 1% sodium hydroxide is added to a supernatant containing maternal blood, whereas a pink colour is obtained with baby blood.

Answer 2.11

a) Urea cycle.
   Organic acidaemia.
   Transient hyperammonaemia of infancy.

b) Plasma amino acids.
   Urine amino acids.
   Urine orotic acid.
   Liver biopsy for specific enzyme analysis.
   Urine organic acids.

Comments There are many inborn errors of metabolism causing hyperammonaemia in the newborn. Commonest of these are various organic acidaemias and deficiencies of the urea cycle enzymes. Hyper-ammonaemia in infants tends to present with symptoms and signs of brain dysfunction, regardless of the cause. There may be hepatomegaly. Respiratory alkalosis may be transiently present during acute exacerbations in the absence of an underlying organic acid disorder. Liver dysfunction may occur. The absence of acidosis in this case makes an organic acidaemia unlikely. Analysis of plasma amino acids, urine amino acids and urine orotic acid is required to define the defect in the urea cycle more accurately.

Ornithine transcarbamylase (OTC) deficiency, an X-linked disorder, is probably the commonest cause; there is no specific amino acid elevation and a high urine orotic acid concentration. The diagnosis can be confirmed by the absence of the enzyme in a liver biopsy.

Answer 2.12

a) QRS axis −80° (i.e. 'superior').

b) Tricuspid atresia.
   Atrio-ventricular (AV) canal defect.

Comments At birth the normal QRS axis lies between +60 and +180°. The marked left axis deviation in the neonatal period shown here is often called a 'superior ' axis, and is commonly due to either tricuspid atresia due to left ventricular dominance or to an AV canal defect due to altered conduction tissue. Left ventricular hypertrophy per se is an uncommon cause of this appearance. In fact this ECG is taken from a baby with Down syndrome with an AV canal defect. In this condition the ECG may later show biatrial and biventricular hypertrophy and a prolonged P–R interval.

Answer 2.13

a) Hereditary fructose intolerance (HFI) due to fructose-1,6-diphosphate aldolase deficiency.

b) Liver biopsy or intestinal mucosal biopsy showing low concentrations of the enzyme fructose-1,6-diphosphate aldolase.

c) A lifelong fructose-free, sucrose-free diet.

Comments The diagnosis of HFI is suggested by the onset of liver disease as soon as fructose is ingested, here with the onset of weaning. It is one of the important causes of acute liver failure in infancy. Renal involvement may cause Fanconi's syndrome. Supportive liver treatment is required on presentation as well as withdrawal of fructose from the diet. Following stabilization and correction of any clotting abnormalities, the diagnosis can be confirmed by liver biopsy or intestinal mucosal biopsy showing low concentrations of the enzyme fructose-1,6-diphosphate aldolase.

Answer 2.14

a) Inadequate fluid therapy.
   Osmotic diuresis due to glycosuria exacerbating dehydration.

b) Increase fluid therapy.
   Reduce water losses (e.g. by transferring to incubator or covering with cling film or similar).
   Reduce concentration of glucose infusion.
   Insulin therapy.

Comments Preterm babies may lose large amounts of fluid, particularly through the skin. This can be exacerbated, as here, by being nursed under a radiant heater and phototherapy units causing large evaporative losses. A high fluid intake needs to be maintained and measures are needed to reduce water losses (e.g. a layer of cling or bubble film overlying the baby and maintaining humidity underneath the film). Hyperglycaemia has many causes in preterm neonates, who frequently have immature glucose homeostasis and a reduced renal threshold for glucose. Glycosuria will increase water losses by causing an osmotic diuresis, as in this case.

Answer 2.15

a) Acquired or secondary lactase deficiency.

b) Lactose-free milk formula.

Comments Secondary carbohydrate intolerance may occur following an episode of acute enteritis, leading to persistence of loose stools. This is most commonly due to acquired or secondary lactase deficiency in the intestinal brush border so that lactose cannot be digested, and much less commonly, a secondary monosaccharide malabsorption. Rotavirus is a common cause of these complications. The diagnosis is suggested by acid stool (normal stool pH > 6.0) due to lactic acid production by bacterial fermentation of unabsorbed lactose. As lactose is a reducing sugar, the excess unabsorbed lactose gives a positive Clinitest reaction (normal stool reducing substances ≤ 0.5%). A short-term lactose-free diet, most commonly with a soy protein-based formula, is appropriate therapy until spontaneous lactase recovery occurs.

Answer 2.16

a) Secondary bacterial infection of the eczema.

b) Systemic antibiotics.
   Liberal use of emollients.
   Topical antiseptic agents.

Comments Secondary infection with bacterial or viral agents must always be considered in a febrile unwell child with eczema or if there is a sudden flare up of the eczema. Staphylococci and streptococci are the bacteria most commonly isolated, and herpes simplex infection must be considered. Treatment is with systemic antibiotics (and acyclovir if herpes simplex infection is suspected), guided by bacterial and viral swabs, and topical antiseptic agents, along with frequent emollients. Topical steroids are added when active infection has subsided.

Answer 2.17

a) Inspissated calcified meconium.
   Intestinal perforation with pneumoperitoneum.

b) Cystic fibrosis.
   Hirschsprung's disease.
   Small bowel atresia.
   Congenital intestinal obstruction.
   Idiopathic meconium ileus.

2

Comments Meconium ileus at birth is the presentation of cystic fibrosis in approximately 10% of cases. This may present either as failure to pass meconium or as passage of sticky inspissated intestinal contents. On occasions this may result in bowel obstruction or intestinal perforation causing meconium peritonitis, sometimes occurring *in utero*, with abdominal radiography occasionally showing calcified meconium as an intra-abdominal high density lesion, typically in the right iliac fossa with associated pneumoperitoneum (as here). A similar appearance may be seen in Hirschsprung's disease, small bowel atresia, congenital intestinal obstruction and idiopathic meconium ileus.

Answer 2.18

a) Cavernous haemangioma of the left posterior chest wall.

b) Spontaneous involution.

Comments Cavernous haemangiomas are more deeply situated than strawberry haemangiomas, and often more extensive. They typically have a phase of growth, which may be rapid, followed eventually by spontaneous resolution. Treatment with systemic or intralesional steroids, interferon, laser or surgical removal is indicated if there is impingement on important structures or interference with functions such as vision. Severe haemorrhage, consumptive coagulopathy or thrombocytopaenia may occur with large lesions.

Answer 2.19

a) Duodenal atresia.

b) Down syndrome.

Comments The typical erect abdominal radiograph of duodenal atresia is shown, with a 'double bubble' gas shadow in the upper abdomen with absence of gas distally. With routine antenatal ultrasound, many cases are now diagnosed prenatally. Postnatally, the condition typically presents with bilious vomiting in the early neonatal period. The same appearance may be seen with severe duodenal stenosis, which is occasionally associated with an annular pancreas, malrotation or a duodenal web. Lesions in the first part of the duodenum may not give the typical 'double bubble' appearance or bilious vomiting. Down syndrome is associated with duodenal atresia.

Answer 2.20

a) Erythema nodosum.

b) Tuberculosis.
   Infection with streptococci, mycoplasma, yersinia or histoplasmosis.
   Sarcoidosis.
   Drugs.
   Inflammatory bowel disease.
   SLE and other vasculitides.
   Idiopathic.

Comments This condition is characterized by painful, red, raised nodules, typically distributed symmetrically over the shins, but also on the upper parts of the legs, buttocks and arms. The lesions usually occur in crops over a 4–6 week period, and are uncommon under the age of six years. A search should be made for a precipitating infection, drug or underlying disease.

Answer 2.21

a) Cherry red spot of the macula.

b) Tay–Sachs disease.
   Niemann–Pick disease.
   Sandhoff's disease.

Comments The cherry red spot is the normal part of the macula in the region of the fovea. The abnormal lighter surround is due to lipid accumulation in retinal ganglion cells in the storage disorders listed above.

Answer 2.22

a) Aspiration pneumonia secondary to a misplaced nasogastric tube in the left main bronchus.

Comments This is always a possibility in a child who is being fed nasogastrically, particularly if there is an associated problem with the bulbar musculature.

Answer 2.23

a) Upturned cardiac apex.
Narrow mediastinum.
Plethoric lung fields.
Diagnosis is transposition of the great arteries.

b) The aorta lies in front of the main pulmonary artery so the pulmonary component of the second heart sound is not heard.

Comments The chest radiograph is a useful investigation in a cyanosed neonate suspected of having cyanotic heart disease. In transposition of the great arteries, there is relative right ventricular predominance because it has to support the systemic circulation, and accompanying plethoric lung fields, in contrast to lesions where there is reduced pulmonary blood flow such as critical pulmonary stenosis or pulmonary atresia. There is a narrow mediastinum ('pedicle') due to loss of the normal relationship of the main pulmonary artery and aorta, with the aorta lying directly in front of the main pulmonary artery.

Answer 2.24

a) Systemic onset juvenile chronic arthritis (JCA).

Comments The characteristic pale pink-red rash, often consisting of discrete (several mm) macules, which occasionally coalesce, is shown in this slide. The rash is typically seen over the trunk, but may occur anywhere, and is fleeting and best seen during febrile episodes. It is present in approximately 90% of patients, and should be actively sought as the other features of systemic onset JCA are not specific. These include fever, hepatosplenomegaly, lymphadenopathy (biopsied lymph nodes may mimic lymphoma, and there may be a leukaemoid blood picture) and anaemia. The arthralgia or arthritis may initially be overlooked because of the overwhelming systemic upset.

Answer 2.25

a) Right chlyothorax secondary to rupture of the thoracic duct.

Comments This is a not infrequent complication following cardiac surgery and can prolong the postoperative course considerably. Diagnosis is made by thoracocentesis, which demonstrates a milky coloured fluid, confirmed as chyle by biochemical analysis and microscopy. Despite thoracocentesis the fluid usually reaccumulates quickly and repeated drainage may deplete calories, protein and lymphocytes, resulting in malnutrition and susceptibility to infection. A medium-chain triglyceride (or low fat) diet supplemented with protein and extra calories should be commenced, with diuretics. In resistant cases, surgery is indicated to ligate the lymph channels (usually the thoracic duct), an alternative being surgical or chemical pleurodesis.

Answer 2.26

a) Presence or absence of testes.

b) Congenital adrenal hyperplasia (CAH) due to 21 α-hydroxylase deficiency (21 α-OHD).
Salt-losing crisis (due to aldosterone deficiency).

Comments In a case of female pseudohermaphroditism (as here) where no gonads are present, the likeliest diagnosis is CAH. 95% of these cases are due to 21 α-OHD, but virilization of females may also occur with two other forms of CAH – 11 β-hydroxylase deficiency and 3 β-hydroxysteroid dehydrogenase deficiency. All these are autosomal recessive disorders with an equal sex incidence. In males, there are often no abnormal clinical findings, though occasionally increased scrotal skin pigmentation may be seen, so presentation is usually with a salt-losing crisis.

Answer 2.27

a) Increased soft tissue swelling in the retropharyngeal space.

b) Retropharyngeal abscess.
Retropharyngeal lymphadenopathy.

Comments This uncommon condition is an important differential diagnosis in a child presenting with an acute onset of stridor with fever. There may be a preceding history of pharyngitis, which is the commonest predisposing condition, and other features are difficulty in swallowing, meningism and systemic upset. Examination (which should only be performed once the airway is secure) often reveals a bulge in the posterior pharyngeal wall. Radiography, as here, is useful in confirming the diagnosis, but again should only be performed if an experienced physician has assessed the airway and found it to be adequate, and must be supervised. The commonest pathogens are *Staphylococcus aureus* and group A haemolytic streptococci.

Answer 2.28

a) Left-sided congenital diaphragmatic hernia.
   Congenital cystic adenomatoid malformation of the lung.
   Pneumatocoeles, as seen in staphylococcal pneumonia.

b) Barium given into the stomach via a nasogastric tube.
   Thoracic CT scan.

Comments When cystic areas are seen on chest radiography in the neonatal period, the differential diagnosis is between a diaphragmatic hernia, congenital cystic adenomatoid malformation of the lung and pneumatocoeles (as seen in staphylococcal pneumonia). Many of these lesions will cause mediastinal shift (as here with the heart displaced into the right hemithorax). A scaphoid abdomen may suggest a congenital diaphragmatic hernia, which is most commonly left sided; if suspected, resuscitation should not be given via a bag and mask device, which will only increase bowel distension within the chest. Although usually involving the stomach, the herniated contents may be other parts of the bowel (as here), and other abdominal viscera with or without the stomach.

Answer 2.29

a) Dermatomyositis – Gottron's papules (collodion patches).

b) Violaceous discoloration (heliotropic appearance) to eyelids.
   Oedema (usually periorbital and extremities).
   Butterfly rash (mimicking SLE).
   Small areas of ulceration or infarcts secondary to small vessel vasculitis.
   Subcutaneous calcification or calcinosis (occasionally intramuscular).
   Telangiectasia.

c) Muscle biopsy.
   Serum creatine kinase.
   EMG.

Comments Dermatomyositis often has an insiduous onset with pain, usually in the muscles, but occasionally arthralgia. Loss of motor skills may be another feature, and muscle weakness eventually develops.

There may be evidence of the skin manifestations already listed. Gottron's papules are scaly red areas over the knuckles, but similar rashes may occur on extensor surfaces of other joints, especially the knees and elbows. Systemic symptoms may be evident. Serum creatine kinase is often raised and EMG shows features of myositis. However, neither of these is diagnostic, so muscle biopsy is required for a definitive diagnosis in the absence of diagnostic clinical features.

Answer 2.30

a) Dilated bronchi or bronchiectasis.
   Lung hyperinflation.
   Left lower lobe collapse/consolidation.

b) Cystic fibrosis.
   Primary ciliary dyskinesia.
   Immunodeficiency.
   Post-pneumonia.
   Gastro-oesophageal reflux.

Comments Whenever bronchiectasis is diagnosed, a search must be made for an underlying abnormality. Cystic fibrosis is the commonest cause, but bronchiectasis may result from primary ciliary dyskinesia, immunodeficiency, gastro-oesophageal reflux (including an isolated H-type fistula) or as a sequelae of severe pneumonia. Specific chest treatment may include prophylactic antibiotics, regular physiotherapy, bronchodilators and inhaled steroids. Chest complications include pneumonia, pneumothorax and, as here, atelectasis secondary to mucus plugging, which is treatable with physiotherapy, mucolytics and plug removal at bronchoscopy.

Answer 2.31

a) Longitudinally aligned areas of radiolucency and increased bone density in the metaphysis.

b) Congenital rubella.

Comments Congenital rubella most commonly arises from maternal rubella infection in the first trimester. Fetal viraemia may result in death or birth of a baby with congenital rubella, which can range from a subclinical disease to severe disease involving multiple target organs and numerous abnormalities. The bone abnormalities shown here are specific for congenital rubella, and differ from those seen in congenital syphilis where there is an accompanying periosteal reaction. The lesions are found in the long bones of the arms and legs, and usually resolve by the age of three months.

Answer 2.32

a) Cigarette burn.

Comments Burns are seen in up to 20% of cases of physical abuse. Of these, cigarette burns typically produce circular punched-out lesions, often with an erythematous edge. The hands and feet are most commonly affected.

Answer 2.33

a) Vaso-occlusive chest crisis.
   Bilateral pneumonia or infective crisis.

b) Analgesia.
   Hydration.
   Ventilatory support.
   Exchange transfusion.
   Antibiotic therapy.

Comments Chest radiography in sickle cell vaso-occlusive chest crisis typically shows bilateral basal atelectasis and/or consolidation (as here) with small volume lungs due to underventilation. It may be difficult to distinguish from an infective crisis, although the latter will often be more focal and not necessarily basal. However, antibiotic treatment is given in both situations. Adequate hydration and analgesia with intravenous opiates, as well as exchange transfusion to lower the sickle cell percentage to less than 20%, are needed. Lung ventilation may be improved with facial continuous positive airway pressure, or failing this, tracheal intubation with positive pressure ventilation.

Answer 2.34

a) Appearances of chronic lung disease/brochopulmonary dysplasia.
   Right upper lobe collapse.

Comments Chronic lung disease arising from ventilation in the first days of life has various definitions, including supplemental oxygen requirement at 28 days, at 36 weeks gestation or on discharge from hospital. Many agents, the most common of which are steroids and diuretics, and other ventilatory modalities e.g. negative pressure, have been tried with varying success to ameliorate the condition. In atypical cases, further investigations need to be performed to exclude a co-existing cardiac condition e.g. left to right shunt or aorto-pulmonary collaterals, gastro-oesophageal reflux, cystic fibrosis, immunodeficiency, lower respiratory tract infection and other conditions as clinically indicated. Any complications, here, the right upper lobe collapse, need to be aggressively treated.

Answer 2.35

a) Bacterial impetigo.

b) *Staphylococcus aureus.*
   Group A haemolytic streptococci.

Comments Bacterial impetigo is a common childhood bacterial skin infection. It typically begins with small bullae, which soon develop characteristic golden crusts. The most commonly affected sites are around the nose and mouth, as here. Treatment is with antibiotics, the route of administration being determined by the extent and severity of the lesions and any systemic upset.

EXAM ANSWERS

ANSWERS – Exam 3
Answer 3.1

a) Chest radiograph.
   Lateral radiograph of the neck.
   Barium swallow.
   Dynamic radiological screening.
   Microlaryngoscopy.
   Echocardiography.

b) Laryngomalacia.
   Acute epiglottis.
   Laryngotracheitis (viral or bacterial).
   Subglottic stenosis (congenital or acquired).
   Foreign body inhalation.
   Subglottic haemangioma.
   Vocal cord palsy (central or peripheral).
   Laryngeal web.
   Allergic oedema of the larynx.
   Laryngeal cleft.
   Vascular ring.
   Haemangioma.
   Laryngeal or bronchogenic cyst.
   Mediastinal tumour.
   Papillomatosis.
   Diphtheria.

3

Comments The commonest cause of stridor from birth is laryngo-malacia, accounting for 60–70% of cases. It presents with inspiratory stridor, which characteristically varies with position and often increases with crying.

If the cause is uncertain or the child has symptoms such as marked respiratory distress or is not thriving, investigations such as a lateral radiograph of the neck, chest radiograph, high KV filter of the neck and barium swallow should be performed to rule out extrinsic compression on the airway.

Subglottic stenosis may present with biphasic stridor, typically being precipitated by concurrent respiratory infection. There is frequently an antecedent history of prolonged intubation. Tracheal stenosis can occur in association with oesophageal atresia and fistulas. Tracheomalacia can be visualized by dynamic screening, which shows collapse of the tracheal wall on expiration. Tracheomalacia can occur with fistulae to the oesophagus or be due to compression by vascular rings.

Rarer causes of extrinsic compression include bronchogenic cysts, which occur mainly in the area of the carina. Thoracic CT is used to delineate the boundaries of this mass.

Vascular rings can be excluded by echocardiography or contrast angiography.

Answer 3.2

a) The diagnosis is Wiskott–Aldrich syndrome, which is associated with both a low platelet cell count and a low platelet volume.

Comments This syndrome tends to present in the first few months of life with bleeding and petechiae. It is an X-linked disorder and predisposes to infection. There is often a low IgM level, an elevated IgA level and a normal IgG level (which includes the subgroups). There is an increased incidence of malignancies of the CNS, especially due to lymphoma.

Answer 3.3

a) Chest radiograph.

Mantoux 10 units of human purified protein derivative (PPD) and 10 units of atypical mycobacterium such as avian PPD intradermally, each one into different forearms.

Biopsy aspiration by fine needle (beware of tracking and fistula formation).

b) Cervical lymphadenopathy due to atypical mycobacterial infection.

Comments The differential diagnosis includes:

- Tuberculosis.
- Cat scratch fever.
- Local dental abscess.
- Kawasaki disease.
- Lymphoma.

Atypical mycobacterium is present in the soil and causes cervical lymphadenopathy, particularly in children under five years of age. The lesion is usually unilateral and does not cause a systemic upset. Kawasaki disease, abscesses and cat scratch fever are all associated with fever. A chest radiograph is useful, along with the Mantoux test, in helping to exlude pulmonary tuberculosis as a cause.

Some authorities recommend total excision of the enlarged lymph nodes; if this is not possible (e.g. if there is a risk of damaging the facial nerve) clarithromycin or erythromycin with ciprofloxacin or erythromycin with cotrimoxazole can be used.

Answer 3.4

a) Cystic fibrosis.

Comments   There is a history of acute onset haematemesis and she has hepatosplenomegaly. She has also been diagnosed for some time as having 'asthma', for which she is receiving inhaled steroids. Clinically she has features of portal hypertension. The normal value for portal venous pressure is 5-10 mm Hg; portal hypertension begins to be seen clinically when it is elevated above 20 mm Hg. Gastro-oesophageal varices and/or ascites can occur.

3

Portal hypertension may be categorized according to the site of the causative lesion as:

- Pre-sinusoidal – either extrahepatic portal vein obstruction such as portal vein thrombosis, damage (e.g. post exchange transfusion via the umbilical vein and/or sepsis) or intrahepatic portal venous obstruction (e.g. congenital hepatic fibrosis, malignant infiltration of the liver).
- Post-sinusoidal – either extra hepatic such as hepatic venous thrombosis (Budd–Chiari) or congestive cardiac failure or intrahepatic (e.g. cirrhosis, which is also sinusoidal).

She also has delayed development of secondary sex characteristics and glycosuria. Her brother died from bowel obstruction, which is a recognized complication of meconium ileus. The most likely cause that would link all these features is cystic fibrosis, hence the diagnostic test would be a sweat test. The 'asthma' diagnosis reflects mild respiratory involvement by cystic fibrosis.

Answer 3.5

a) The three features are encephalopathy, fever and dysentery.

b) Infection.
   Post-infectious disease.
   Mass lesion.
   Metabolic disorder.
   Acute demyelinating disorder.

Toxic agent.
Status epilepticus.

Comments   The history of fever, dysentery and encephalopathy in a previously well child suggests in this case an infective cause and Shigella was the causative bacterial pathogen. Hyponatraemia and low WCC are common in Shigella encephalopathy. The PT is often slightly prolonged. Other complications caused by this organism include septicaemia, haemolytic uraemic syndrome, meningitis, pneumonia and dehydration. Acute encephalopathy is also caused by infection with viruses, fungi, chlamydia, mycoplasma and parasitic agents.

Post-infectious diseases such as Guillain–Barré syndrome, brain stem encephalitis and acute cerebellar ataxia are excluded as no focal neurology is seen. Similarly, a mass lesion such as a tumour is unlikely as this will often cause focal signs or signs of raised intracranial pressure. Here there is no localized neurological deficit and the fundus appears normal.

Metabolic causes include hypoglycaemia, uraemia, inborn errors of metabolism and hepatic disorders. In this case, however, the ammonia is not elevated as it is in Reye's syndrome, the bilirubin is within normal limits and the PT (a very sensitive indicator of liver disease) is also normal. The glucose is 8 mmol/l, which is normal. Many metabolic disorders are also associated with an acidosis, but here the pH is 7.44.

Acute demyelinating disorders such as acute multiple sclerosis are a rare cause of encephalopathy and the majority of cases occur in adults. Only 5% of cases of multiple sclerosis are seen in the under 15s with the commonest presentation being a visual disturbance. Generally, the course of multiple sclerosis is intermittent relapses and recovery with increasing residual neurological deficits after each relapse.

Toxic agents are excluded by the toxicology screen and status epilepticus is clearly not the cause.

Answer 3.6

a)   There is an alkalosis and hypochloraemia. Persistent vomiting leads to a loss of chloride ions as well as hydrogen ions causing alkalosis. The kidney tries to conserve hydrogen ions at the expense of potassium, which is lost in the urine; hence the urine is alkalotic and has a relatively high concentration of potassium.

? Acidic urine

b)   These results suggest a diagnosis of congenital hypertrophic pyloric stenosis.

Answer 3.7

a) The features are of failure to thrive with elevated renal function markers and an increased blood pressure suggesting renal failure. There is hyperkalaemic acidosis, which is a common feature of acute renal failure.

Comments   Causes include congenital renal failure due to conditions such as polycystic renal disease, other dysplastic conditions or, as he is a boy, posterior urethral valves.

Answer 3.8

a) Bartter's syndrome.

Comments   She has a picture of failure to thrive with a normal blood pressure and hypokalaemic alkalosis. This is due to hyperaldosteronism caused by juxtaglomerular hyperplasia. Treatment is with potassium supplements and anti-inflammatory agents such as indomethacin. This biochemical profile could also be seen in older children as a result of laxative abuse.

Answer 3.9

a) Congenital adrenal hyperplasia (CAH), which is inherited in an autosomal recessive fashion, the commonest form being due to 21-α hydroxylase deficiency.

Comments   The potassium is elevated as there is a lack of aldosterone, which facilitates sodium and potassium exchange in the kidneys. Potassium excretion occurs largely in the distal section of the collecting duct.

Answer 3.10

a) This child has hypernatraemic dehydration and requires careful rehydration. If her circulation is insufficient and she is showing signs of shock, attention must be paid to her airway, breathing and circulation, in that order. If her circulatory parameters are within normal limits and she is not showing signs of shock, correction of her volume deficit should take place gradually, with 2–4 hourly repeated reassessment of her electrolyte status. As a rule of thumb the plasma sodium should decrease by about 1–2 mmol per litre per hour.

Answer 3.11

a) Coarctation of the aorta.

b) DiGeorge syndrome.

Comments The child presents with a difference between his right arm and all the other limb blood pressure measurements, which is indicative of an obstruction such as coarctation of the aorta. Biochemically he is acidotic and has elevated renal function markers, probably from insufficient renal perfusion. The total calcium is low and with the presence of a heart lesion such as coarctation of the aorota, this suggests DiGeorge syndrome. T-cell function may be affected because this condition is associated with thymic aplasia as well as an absence of parathyroid glands (hence hypocalcaemia). Therefore only irradiated CMV-negative blood should be given to this child as there is a distinct possibility that graft versus host syndrome could arise from residual white cells in transfused blood overwhelming the child's poor immune defence.

Answer 3.12

a) These features fit the social development of a two-year-old. At this age he would tend to be clingy to his parent and be possessive of his toys.

Answer 3.13

a) Alport's syndrome.

Comments This is characterized by deafness and the development of a glomerulonephritis. It is inherited in an autosomal X-linked manner.

Answer 3.14

a) von Willebrand's disease.

	Haemophilia	von Willebrand's disease	Vitamin K deficiency
Bleeding time	Normal	Increased	Normal
PT	Normal	Normal	Increased
APPT	Increased	Increased	Normal
VIII:c	Decreased	Decreased	Normal
VIII:vWF	Normal	Absent/very low	Normal

Comments This child shows a normal PT, abnormal APTT and prolonged bleeding time. This suggests that he has von Willebrand's disease (see table below). The prolonged bleeding time arises as von

Willebrand's factor is involved in platelet adhesion to the endothelium. If the level is less than 1% severe bleeding episodes with joint bleeding occurs. Less than 5% is associated with marked blood loss after minor trauma.

Answer 3.15

a) Vitamin D dependent rickets.
Vitamin D malabsorption.
Liver disease.
Renal phosphate leak.

Comments The serum calcium is low, but the serum phosphate is only slightly reduced. This makes malabsorption or an increased renal leak (e.g. hypophosphataemic or vitamin D resistant rickets) of phosphate unlikely. Lack of response to vitamin D may be due to poor compliance, but this is not implied in the question. Other causes may be poor absorption as seen in small bowel and liver disease, reduced hepatic conversion to 25(OH) vitamin D, reduced kidney conversion to $1,25(OH)_2D$ or lack of end-organ response to $1,25(OH)_2D$. The two latter causes are often referred to as vitamin D dependent rickets types I and II respectively, and are the most likely causes in this case due to only slightly reduced serum phosphate. Large doses of vitamin D_2 or $1,25(OH)_2D$ should be tried if this is suspected.

Answer 3.16

a) A left-sided diaphragmatic hernia.

Comments Diaphragmatic hernias are commoner on the left than right and may be associated with pulmonary hypoplasia. The majority of children with diaphragmatic hernias are diagnosed antenatally, but in those children in whom the upward progression occurs after the last routine scan at 12–16 weeks there may be a delay in diagnosis. These children may present on the ward with tachypnoea and an absence of breath sounds on auscultation on the affected side. A chest radiograph in these cases is all revealing!

Answer 3.17

a) *Plasmodium vivax* in erythrocytes.

Comments The blood films shown tend to be very classical in appearance. The common topics include microangiopathic anaemia as seen in haemolytic uraemic syndrome, target cells, Burr cells, sickle cell cells. A pale film with a microcytic anaemia which does not respond to iron treatment is often due to thalassaemia.

3

Answer 3.18

a) Giant cystic hygroma.

b) Overall the prognosis is poor as there is a compression of the airway.

Comments Compression of the airway may be associated with intrathoracic extension with obstruction of thoracic vessels leading to cardiovascular compromise. Resection may provide relief only temporarily as this lesion has a tendency to recur.

Answer 3.19

a) Kasai operation.

b) Extrahepatic biliary atresia.

Comments This operation involves forming a roux-en-Y, with the small bowel being brought up to where the porta hepatis should be. Satisfactory drainage of the liver can then result.

Answer 3.20

a) Epidermolysis bullosa.

b) Contractures and loss of motility.
Hand function may be lost owing to fusion of fingers, and the same process occurs with the toes.
Increased incidence of dermal malignancies such as small cell carcinomas.

Answer 3.21

a) Treacher–Collins syndrome.

b) The associated anomalies include antimongoloid slanting palpebral fissures, hypoplasia of the malar bones, which may involve a cleft in the zygomatic bones, mandibular hypoplasia, coloboma of the lower lid, malformation of the pinna and cleft palate. Prenatal diagnosis is possible.

Answer 3.22

a) Pleural effusions bilaterally.
Soft tissue oedema.
Atrial and ventricular pacing wire.
A central mediastinal drain.

Comments   All the features should be stated in the answer. In looking at the chest radiograph the candidate must apply his or her routine procedure for analysing it as would be done in clinical practice. Look at the orientation of the film, then inspect the soft tissue and bony structures. Make sure there are no fractures or radiological evidence of rickets fractures or even an osteosarcoma involving the humeral head. Check that there are no butterfly vertebrae. Look for all the tubes and foreign materials within the picture and think of where that two-dimensional object may be located and why. Then look at the cardiac borders and the distinguishing characteristics of its borders. Do not forget to look behind the heart as in lingual collapse and to check that the right heart border is not obscured, as in right middle lobe pneumonia. Rotate the picture through 90° so that the mind's eye is less drawn to the heart and look carefully at the lung fields. Is there vascular pruning as in pulmonary hypertension, or a lobar emphysema, or a marked difference between the volume of the right and left lungs with expiration, indicating the presence of an inhaled foreign body.

A careful systematic approach will give much of the required information.

3

Answer 3.23

a)   This child has chickenpox.

b)   As this is happening outside the neonatal period there is no appreciably increased risk and passive immunization in this otherwise healthy child is not necessary.

Answer 3.24

a)   Target cells.

Comments   Target cells are seen in haemoglobinopathies such as sickle cell, HbSC (a haemoglobinopathy in which HbS and HbC are present in the same molecule), thalassaemia, iron deficiency anaemia, lead poisoning and liver disease and post-splenectomy.

Answer 3.25

a)   This chest radiograph shows an intubated patient who has a tension pneumothorax on the right. He has a ligated ductus arteriosus and evidence of previous thoracic surgery, as evidenced by displaced ribs on left and right. The stomach is also distended.

Answer 3.26

a) She has alopecia areata, which is associated with autoimmune disease.

Comments There is an increased association of alopecia areata with autoantibodies, and atopic children have a higher incidence of this condition. There may be a family history.

Answer 3.27

a) Familial microcephaly in both child and father!

Comments There is a form of autosomal recessive microcephaly, which is associated with marked developmental delay.

Answer 3.28

a) Poland's anomaly with bilateral absence of pectoralis minor.

Comments Poland's anomaly is usually associated with unilateral absence of pectoralis major and with unilateral syndactyly.

Answer 3.29

a) Micrognathia.
   Cleft palate.
   Upper airway obstruction.

Comments This child has Pierre-Robin sequence. This is a developmental anomaly arising *in utero* and comprises micrognathia, often with a cleft palate owing to the relatively normal tongue pushing upward within the narrower than expected buccal cavity hindering fusion of the bony processes forming the hard palate. Upper airway obstruction can be caused by the tongue being displaced posteriorly, which can lead to cor pulmonale.

Answer 3.30

a) Marfan syndrome. This picture illustrates arachnodactyly of the toes!

Comments Marfan syndrome is associated with tall stature, kyphoscoliosis, lens displacement, hyperextensibility and dilatation with or without dissecting aneursym of the aorta. Less common cardiovascular involvement includes aortic and mitral valve prolapse.

Answer 3.31

a) This child has prune belly syndrome.

Comments This arises because *in utero* there is megaureter, which distends the anterior abdominal muscular wall. Renal damage may occur and can produce oligohydramnios and marked contractures.

Answer 3.32

a) There is a filling defect in the descending colon due to stricture formation.

Comments It is vital that studies are performed before reanastomosis to ensure patency, not only distally to the gut lumen, but also proximally.

Answer 3.33

a) Extra corporeal membrane oxygenation (ECMO) with an internal right carotid cannula going into the arch of the aorta and a larger bore cannula going into the right atrium via the right internal jugular vein.

Comments There is a widespread opacification of both lungs, which is commonly seen in these children. There is an air bronchogram in the right upper zone.

Answer 3.34

a) Gaucher's disease.

Comments Foam cells are seen in this bone marrow, which suggests the diagnosis. Bone marrow studies tend to show leukaemias, infiltrates from other neoplasias such as neuroblastomas or foam cells. Bone marrow slides can also be used to show aplastic anaemia in the exam.

Answer 3.35

a) Cavernous sinus thrombosis.
   Sinusitis.
   Cerebral abscess.
   Subdural collection.
   Meningitis.

EXAM ANSWERS

1
2
3
4
5
6

ANSWERS - Exam 4

Answer 4.1

a) As he is showing neurological complications of hypertension, this must be dealt with first after ensuring that his airway, breathing and circulation are all satisfactory.

b) Investigations include bone marrow (which can show diffuse marrow infiltration of malignant cells), bone scan (which can show multiple lytic lesions), MIBG scan (even more sensitive than bone scan at picking up active centres) and liver biopsy (which can show liver infiltration). Urinary catecholamines and abdominal and thoracic CT may also be useful in determining the extent of the disease.

Comments This is a child who presents with an altered level of consciousness, who has a facial palsy and an abdominal mass. The most likely cause of all these features is a neuroblastoma secreting catecholamines. A less likely diagnosis is Wilms' tumour as it does not generally cause hypertension. It is, however, associated with hemi-hypertrophy.

Answer 4.2

a) This child appears to have episodic periods of hypertension, calcium deposition in his kidneys and mood changes. All these features can be explained by MEN type II.

b) This condition also comprises hyperparathyroidism leading to hypercalcaemia and episodic hypertension owing to phaeochromocytoma. Adrenal medullary hyperplasia is also seen. His psychological disturbance may be caused by his hypercalcaemia. There may also be malignancy of the C cells of the thyroid in MEN type II.

Answer 4.3

a) This shows a narrow chest with flaring of the lower ribs and short horizontal ribs. The costochondral junctions are expanded and the clavicles are set high.

b) Asphyxiating thoracic dystrophy (Jeune's syndrome).
Thanatophoric dwarfism.
Achondrogenesis.
Homozygous achondroplasia.
Chondoectodermal dystrophy (Ellis–van Creveld syndrome).

4

Comments Thanatophoric dwarfism, homozygous achondroplastic dwarfism and achondrogenesis are rapidly fatal conditions. Both parents do not have a past medical history, which is likely to exclude homozygous achondroplasia as a cause.

Achondrogenesis results in a poorly ossified skull, with short ribs and severe micromelia. In one form the ribs are not fractured, but in all cases death occurs shortly after birth. Thanatophoric dysplasia results in short limbs, flat vertebrae, a large head and low nasal bridge with narrow shortened ribs as its main features. The head is large and can produce problems with vaginal delivery; death occurs within the first few weeks of life due to respiratory insufficiency.

Ellis–van Creveld syndrome has other notable features such as disproportionate short limbs, with polydactyly, hypoplastic nails, neonatal teeth, short upper lip and defects in the alveolar ridge. About 50% of cases have an associated cardiac lesion, the commonest being an atrioseptal defect. It is inherited in an autosomal recessive fashion.

This child has asphyxiating thoracic dystrophy, which is due to disordered growth at the costochrondral junctions and a failure of ossification of the ribs. The key components are short stature and short ribs and on radiography the pelvis has a square contour with inferior bony protrusions into the sciatic notch and acetabulum producing the 'trident sign'. There may be renal involvement with tubular dysplasia, which can lead to renal failure. It occurs sporadically as well as by autosomal recessive inheritance.

Answer 4.4

a) Septo-optic dysplasia.

Comments This child has a conjugated hyperbilirubinaemia due to an intrahepatic pathology. The causes of intrahepatic disorders in infancy can be divided into the following categories:

- Infective.
- Inherited conditions such as inborn errors of metabolism.
- Chromosomal abnormalities and genetic conditions.
- Drugs.
- Endocrine.

Infective causes include bacteria such as *Escherichia coli* and Listeria. Other bacteria causing septicaemia can also produce a hepatitis. Agents such as cytomegalovirus, rubella, chickenpox, varicella zoster, echovirus, rheovirus, hepatitis A and B, and toxoplasmosis can cause hepatic disturbances ranging from a minor alteration in liver function tests to full-blown liver failure.

Metabolic causes include galactosaemia, fructosaemia, cystic fibrosis, tyrosinaemia, α-1-antitrypsin deficiency, Gaucher's disease, Zellweger syndrome and Dubin–Johnson syndrome. The glucose is normal and the urine does not contain reducing substances or amino acids. Gaucher's disease at this age would cause splenomegaly as an associated feature. The phenotype for α-1-antitrypsin is normal and Dublin–Johnson syndrome is usually associated with a positive family history.

The features of Down's syndrome, Edwards' or Patau's syndrome are not seen in this case. Alagille syndrome is associated with intrahepatic biliary hypoplasia and also characteristic facies, vertebral abnormalities such as butterfly vertebral bodies and posterior embryotoxon on fundoscopy.

Drugs such as frusemide, erythromycin, chloramphenicol and chloral hydrate have all been implicated in causing liver disease. Neonates who have required umbilical venous catherization are exposed to the risk of the catheter becoming placed into a portal vein branch off the inferior vena cava, which can lead to thrombosis and focal necrosis.

The endocrine group of causes include hypoparathyroidism, hypothyroidism, hypoadrenalism, diabetes inspidus and hypopituitarism. Of these hypopituitarism is the most likely diagnosis as he has small genitalia. The key feature that helps to make the full diagnosis is the presence of pale discs on fundoscopy. This suggests septo-optic dysplasia. This condition comprises absence of the septum pellucidum, optic nerve hypoplasia, variable degrees of hypopituitarism and small genitalia.

Answer 4.5

a) Fanconi's anaemia.

Comments The causes of a pancytopenia with organomegaly and an abnormal bone marrow include leukaemia and storage conditions such as Gaucher's disease. Pancytopenia, organomegaly and a normal bone marrow may be due to lymphoma or hypersplenism. In pancytopenias where there is no organomegaly, an abnormal bone marrow examination would tend to be due to leukaemia, whereas a hypocellular marrow means that there is an aplastic anaemia. Aplastic anaemia may be acquired or congential in orgin. Acquired causes arise from exposure to radiation, to drugs such as cytotoxic drugs or benzene and to viruses such as Ebstein–Barr virus, parvovirus or HIV. Inherited causes are:

- Schwachmann–Diamond syndrome.
- Dyskeratosis congenita.
- Fanconi's anaemia.

Pancytopenia can also be seen in Down's, Dubowitz's and Seckel's syndromes.

This girl is dysmorphic and has abnormal hands, café au lait patches, a heart lesion, cardiac enlargement on chest radiography and a pancytopenia. There is also consanguinity in this family. Schwachmann–Diamond syndrome is due to an insufficiency of exocrine pancreatic secretions and neutropaenia. Features are short stature, failure to thrive, malabsorption and steatorrhoea. Over 40% of cases have typical metaphyseal dysostosis.

Dyskeratosis results in dermal pigmentation, delay in development, nail dystrophy, short stature, oesophageal diverticula, telangiectasia and abnormal dentition. It is an X-linked condition. There is an association with chromosomal breaks that are characteristic of Fanconi's anaemia in only 10% of cases.

Fanconi's anaemia is typified by abnormal chromosomal breakages. Clinical features are short stature and abnormalities of the upper limbs varying from absent or abnormal thumbs to absent radii and micromelia. Syndactyly may also be seen. The gonads may be small and the testes abnormal. There may be micropenis and hysplia and in females, there may be abnormal development of the vagina, uterus and ovaries. Skeletal abnormalities are common and include spina bifida, abnormal ribs and vertebral anomalies. There may be a global developmental delay. The head may be microcephalic and there may be micrognathia and/or hydrocephalus. The cardiac malformations include PDA, VSD, ASD, tetralogy of Fallot (TOF) suggested by the boot shape and PS. There may also be deafness.

Answer 4.6

a) Pseudo-Bartter's syndrome.

Comments In this case pseudo-Bartter's syndrome is caused by cystic fibrosis, which produces an increased sodium loss through excessive sweat (owing to a defect in the sodium chloride/sodium exchange in the sweat glands). To ameliorate the sweat loss of sodium there is intense reabsorption in the renal tubules and with the associated contraction in extracellular circulation there is stimulation of the production of the angiotensin and so elevated levels of aldosterone. In Bartter's syndrome there is a normal sweat profile and the renal clearances of electrolytes are abnormal.

Other causes of a metabolic alkalosis in association with low electrolyte levels include abuse of chlorothiazide diuretics, pyloric stenosis, chloride-losing nephropathy and gastric drainage without appropriate electrolyte replacement. Laxative abuse can also be a cause

Answer 4.7
a) This is the characteristic picture seen in poisoning with ethylene glycol.

Comments This is metabolized to harmful products mediated by alcohol dehydrogenase. The treatment is to inhibit this enzyme competitively by using ethanol, aiming to achieve blood levels of 100 mg/dl. Co-factors such as thiamine and pyridoxine tend to be given as well. In some cases haemodialysis has been used.

Answer 4.8
a) 21-α hydroxylase assay.
   Urea and electrolyte measurements.

Comments This may be a salt losing 21-hydroxylase deficiency. This deficiency accounts for 90% of cases of congenital adrenal hyperplasia. These infants may develop raised serum potassium and hyponatraemia with elevated urinary sodium values. If this proved normal, the possibility of 11-β hydroxylase deficiency should be investigated. This may give rise to hypertension.

Answer 4.9
a) Bilateral renal artery stenosis.

Comments Causes of systemic hypertension include:

- Renal causes – acute glomerulonephritis, chronic glomerulonephritis, chronic pyelonephritis, polycystic kidneys, Wilms' tumour, vasculitides such as SLE.
- Endocrine causes – phaeochromocytoma, adrenogenital syndrome, Cushing's disease, primary hyperaldosteronism, hyperthyroidism.
- Cardiovascular causes – coarctation of the aorta, renal artery stenosis, renal artery or renal venous thrombosis.
- Medication – steroids or ACTH.

The commonest cause of hypertension in infancy is coarctation of the aorta. Renal causes such as renal artery stenosis, renal vessel thrombosis and congenital renal abnormalities are the next most common cause. His features include hypertension, but the four limb blood pressure measurements are normal, urine cultures are negative, there is no evidence of a nephritis or renal vessel thrombosis as the biochemical urinalysis has been clear, DMSA is normal and renal ultrasound is normal. He does have small abdominal vessels on ultrasound and an elevated renin level. This is suggestive of bilateral renal artery stenosis as the kidneys do not differ in size from each other as would be seen in renal parenchymal disease or unilateral renal artery stenosis. Normal urinalysis is not seen in glomerulonephritis, renal vein thrombosis and pyelonephritis.

In Conn's syndrome, renal primary hyperaldosteronism, there is an elevated sodium (greater than 140 mmol/l) and a low potassium (usually less than 3 mmol/l).

Answer 4.10

a) This lesion is due to compression on the optic chiasm. This is clasically caused by craniopharyngioma or ituitary tumour.

b) Craniopharyngioma, pituitary tumour or other masses such as neurofibroma or tubers as in tuberous sclerosis.

Answer 4.11

a) This girl has C1 esterase inhibitor deficiency.

Comments   This protein inhibits the activated form of C1 as well as other proteins such as kallikrein and plasmin. In an attack unrestrained C1 cleaves C4 and C2. The level of C1 esterase can be measured directly to confirm the diagnosis.

Answer 4.12

a) The ability to draw a square starts at 4.5 years, a circle at 3 and a triangle at 5.5 years.

Answer 4.13

a) Bernard–Soulier disease.

Comments   The platelet aggregation response is used to differentiate thrombasthenia (Glanzmann's syndrome), which is due to platelet membrane abnormalities, from Bernard–Soulier disease in which there is a defect in the platelet receptors as shown in the table opposite.

	ADP	Adrenaline	Ristocetin	Collagen
Glanzmann's syndrome	Abn	Abn	Abn/N	Abn
Bernard–Soulier disease	N	N	Abn	N
Cyclo-oxygenase/ thromboxane synthetase deficiency or aspirin	N	Abn	N	Abn
Abn, abnormal; N, normal				

Answer 4.14

a) There is a step-up in saturation at the atrial level suggesting an inter-atrial connexion.

b) As the atrial pressure is normal this would tend to rule out ostium primum as the lesion as involvement of the mitral valve is very common in this condition; hence the answer is atrial secundum defect.

Answer 4.15

a) This child has maple syrup urine disease.

Comments This is an inheritable autosomal recessive condition due to a deficiency in ketoacid decarboxylase, which can be assayed in white cells or from fibroblast culture. Other clinical features include feeding difficulties, respiratory distress, and neurological complications such as fitting, spasticity and coma.

Answer 4.16

a) There is air under the diaphragm.

Comments Look below as well as above the diaphragm on the chest radiograph!

Answer 4.17

a) Fetal alcohol syndrome.

Comments The characteristic features seen in this picture are mild to moderate microcephaly, smooth philtrum, maxillary hypoplasia and a smooth upper lip. Other features of this condition include intrauterine growth retardation, failure to thrive after birth and low IQ.

Answer 4.18

a) This child had a failed ventouse extraction and has the marks of the blades of the forceps, which assisted in his delivery.

Comments Complications of ventouse extraction can include scalping (!) and the introduction of infection, which can pass via bridging veins to the dura. Haemorrhage can be significant in severe injuries sustained in this manner.

Answer 4.19

a) This child has PICA.

Comments There is stippling throughout the intraluminal contents of the bowel. The abdominal radiograph must be approached systematically. Inspect the bony and soft tissues structures. Determine the location of the stomach by looking for the gas bubble. A double bubble obviously means trouble! See that there is a complete sacrum and carefully check the continuity of the pelvis. Odd soft tissue shadowing within the abdomen may be due to a mass (e.g. intussusception) or neoplasm (e.g. Wilms' tumour). Relate the findings to the clinical information given. Free air under the diaphragm either means that there is perforation of a viscus or that air has been introduced into the abdomen (e.g. an open wound following trauma).

Answer 4.20

a) This lesion is an ashleaf patch.

Comments Ashleaf patches are seen in tuberous sclerosis. Other associated dermatological conditions include fibroangiomatous lesions, café au lait patches, fibromatous plaques and nodules.

Answer 4.21

a) This child has gastroschisis.

Comments This is due to a complete defect in all the anterior abdominal layers.

Answer 4.22

a) A bite mark. (This arose from a dispute with another child on the ward over ownership of the empty tin he is holding!)

Comments Non-accidental injuries commonly occur in the picture presentation section of the exam. Be familiar with the appearance of bite marks, marks made by cigarette burns, the appearance of pinch marks on the face and limbs, the bruises caused by caning, torn frenula and bruises occuring in peculiar sites such as on the pinna, especially in young children, and particularly infants.

Answer 4.23

a) There is marked dilation of the lateral and temporal ventricles with organized clot in the right ventricle and newer haemorrhage in the other.

Comments The candidate should make him or herself familiar with cranial ultrasound scans, as they are increasingly common in the exam.

Answer 4.24

a) He has kwashiorkor.

Comments This child has had prolonged protein deficiency causing oedema, friable depigmented hair, hepatomegaly, growth retardation, muscle wasting, poor appetite and (usually) irritability. (The child pictured above is obviously getting better as he is laughing while filling his nappy!)

Answer 4.25

a) An H-type tracheo-oesophageal fistula.

Comments This slide shows contrast material revealing the H fistula. This may be associated with recurrent chest infections and needs surgical intervention.

Answer 4.26

a) There is a marked scoliosis, which has an S shape.

Comments The complications of this condition include restrictive pulmonary disease and cor pulmonale. Recurrent aspiration can also occur. Developmental delay may also be seen in such severe cases as mobility is greatly reduced.

Answer 4.27

a) There is a lung abscess.

Comments   There is a well-demarcated spherical object, which is due to a walled abscess. This implies that it is not recently aquired as an inflammatory reaction has occurred. This may be caused by a number of organisms such as *Mycobacterium tuberculosis*, staphylococci and Klebsiella.

Answer 4.28

a) A right haemothorax.

Comments   As this is a life-threatening event he needs attention to his airway, ventilation and circulation. Get experienced help as soon as possible. He needs 100% oxygen (if inadequately ventilating then bag mask ventilation or intubation, preferably by an anaesthetist) with two large bore canulae with volume replacement to hand and a chest drain on the side of the haemothorax. With this amount of damage there may be underlying pulmonary contusion and close monitoring is required.

Answer 4.29

a) This child has cervical tuberculosis.

Comments   Atypical mycobacterial infections do not often form draining sinuses.

Answer 4.30

a) This child has hydrocephalus and a lower myelocele.

Comments   If this child is seen as a short case remember to determine his or her sphincter control and mobility and *always ask to plot head circumference, height and weight.*

Answer 4.31

a) This child has Henoch–Schönlein purpura.

Comments   There is an associated glomerulonephritis and a high incidence of intussusception. Melaena may also occur.

Answer 4.32

a) This radiograph shows an intubated patient with a tension pneumothorax on the right, a ligated ductus arteriosus, previous surgery (as evidenced by the rib displacement on the left and right sides) and a distended stomach.

Answer 4.33

a) It shows an extensive purpuric rash with patches of ecchymoses.

b) Meningococcaemia.

Comments This child is shocked and the most likely diagnosis in the UK is meningococcaemia.

Answer 4.34

a) Acanthocytes.

Comments Acanthocytes are seen in severe starvation, anorexia nervosa, hepatocellular disease and abetalipoproteinaemia. In abetalipoproteinaemia (beloved subject of examiners!) there is a progessive ataxia, absence of chylomicrons, retinitis pigmentosa and fat malabsorption. It is due to the failure of synthesis or secretion of lipoproteins.

Answer 4.35

a) There is marked tracheal deviation to the left with the appearance of a soft tissue mass pushing it away.

Comments Tracheal deviation may be due to extrinsic compressive forces (as seen in this radiograph), which may be due to neoplasia and can be seen with marked lymphadenopathy or haemorrhage into soft tissue.

EXAM
ANSWERS

1

2

3

4

5

6

Answer 5.1

a) 17-hydroxyprogesterone.
   Plasma renin activity – a sensitive assessment of mineralocorticoid function.
   Karyotype.
   Pelvic ultrasound.
   Urinary steroid profile.
   Plasma oestradiol assay.
   GnRH test.

b) Non salt-wasting late-onset 21-hydroxylase congenital adrenal hyperplasia (CAH).

c) Hydrocortisone and fludrocortisone steroid replacement therapy.
   Clitoral reduction and perineal reconstruction (if necessary).
   Psychological support.
   Education and genetic counselling.

Comments   This girl presents with advanced, but disordered (disso-nant) puberty, which accounts for her tall stature. The timing of puberty has undoubtedly been premature and the pubertal sequence abnormal. For this degree of pubic and axillary hair, the absence of breast changes is abnormal. This dissonance suggests an endocrinopathy. Furthermore, this pattern of development suggests that the precocious puberty is gonadotrophin independent. The marked accompanying virilization indicates an adrenal focus of pathology.

Adrenal dysfunction is indicated by the elevated ACTH concentration in the absence of disordered cortisol secretion. Androstenedione eleva-tion indicates increased androgen activity, suggesting a steroid synthetic pathway block. The most common cause is 21-hydroxylase deficient CAH (21-OH CAH). This was demonstrated by an elevated 17-hydroxy-progesterone level and characteristic urinary steroid profile.

Although classical salt-losing 21-OH CAH is more frequently encoun-tered, non salt-losing or late-onset presentation disease may occur. The key is the determination of dissonant precocious puberty with evi-dence of adrenal abnormality. Adequate steroid replacement will allow the sequence of pubertal changes to normalise with breast develop-ment and a reduction in acne. Clitoral reduction is performed, together with careful examination of the external and internal female sexual tract to identify other structural abnormalities. Psychological therapy is vital to temper the features of precocious puberty as well as the effects of surgery and the impact of the diagnosis itself. Subfertil-ity is common due to the association with polycystic ovary disease.

Despite the maternal history of subfertility both mother and sibling were normal on testing.

Answer 5.2

a) Anti dsDNA autoantibodies (anti-dsDNA).
Antinuclear antibodies (ANA).
Anticardiolipin antibodies.
Anti-neutrophil cystoplasmic antibodies (ANCA).
Bone marrow aspirate.
Renal biopsy.
CNS imaging.

b) Systemic lupus erythematosis.

c) Methylprednisolone. ✓
Cyclophosphamide. ✓
Azathioprine.
Plasmapheresis. ✓
General supportive care. ✓

Comments   This boy presents with a fever without a focus. Furthermore, he demonstrates significant renal impairment and myelosuppression. A streptococcal infection would initially fit with some of the clinical features, but the ASOT and bacteriology studies are negative. The greatly elevated ESR with a normal CRP suggests either an atypical infection or an autoimmune disorder. The erythema multiforme would fit either, but has a vasculitic component. Kawasaki disease is excluded on the basis of the thrombocytopenia and neutropenia, which do not occur in this disorder. Haematological malignancy remains in the differential diagnosis, but may be excluded on the bone marrow biopsy. Other vasculitides are possible (e.g. polyarteritis, Wegener's granulomatosis), but this constellation of features favours the diagnosis of SLE.

The diagnosis may be confirmed by autoimmune serology, particularly the anti-dsDNA. The vasculitic component may result from thromboses due to circulating anticardiolipin antibodies, which cause the antiphospholipid syndrome. ANCA antibodies are non-specific and are identified in vasculitides such as Kawasaki disease, SLE and Wegener's granulomatosis. In this case, lupus nephritis is a complication, as shown by the proteinuria, biochemical renal impairment and depressed complement levels. His disorientation may be a feature of his fever or a sign of impending cerebral lupus.

Treatment is a combination of general supportive care and glucocorticosteroids. Immunosuppressives such as cyclophosphamide are often necessary in cases of nephritis, although myelosuppression is a relative contraindication. The prognosis is variable, with 80–90% five-year survival rate. Approximately 15% of survivors are cured. Renal involvement occurs in 80% with cerebral lupus and persists in 40–50% of sufferers. Death is usually due to infective complications.

Answer 5.3

a) Congenital sepsis.

b) Coxsackie virus.

c) General supportive care.

Comments The infant, born at a preterm gestation but appropriate weight, manifests respiratory, haemodynamic and neurological dysfunction. The preterm passage of meconium is often a sign of perinatal sepsis, particularly listeriosis. Meconium aspiration could potentially cause the clinical and radiological features, but no evidence of aspiration was noted on intubation, thus reducing the likelihood of this complication. However, respiratory failure was noted, which was then exacerbated by the pulmonary haemorrhage, a rare complication but one associated with sepsis. The haemorrhage and increase in mechanical ventilation can account for the radiological features, including the air leak. There is no suggestion of a primary cardiac or pulmonary disease.

The diagnosis of perinatal sepsis is supported by the thrombocytopenia, neutropenia and disseminated coagulopathy. Although bacteriological cultures are sterile, further acute inflammatory markers may be helpful to discriminate between bacterial and viral causes. The CSF result is suggestive of a viral meningitis picture. Therefore all the above can be explained by an overwhelming viraemic illness.

The maternal illness before delivery was similar to pleurodynia (Bornholm disease) which is a coxsackie virus infection causing severe chest pain with extreme thoracic tenderness. The diagnosis was confirmed by coxsackie B2 isolated from the fetal lung at autopsy.

Coxsackie and other enteroviruses can be transmitted transplacentally. Maternal infection may appear trivial. These viruses have been implicated in still birth and miscarriage. Perinatal enteroviral disease may be predominantly meningoencephalitic or present as an overwhelming disseminated viraemia. Other presentations include hepatitis, pancreatitis and necrotizing enterocolitis. Treatment, if possible, is supportive.

5

Answer 5.4

a) Postviral chronic fatigue syndrome (PVCFS).

b) Debatable!! The effects of immune stimulation, possibly with persistent infection, alters endogenous endorphin release, which affects neural biochemistry. This in turn has an effect on the psyche, therefore causing behavioural problems.

c) Multidisciplinary approach involving:

- Paediatrician – to exclude other diseases and positively diagnose PVCFS.
- Psychologist – to provide support to the child and family, explore areas of family tension and aid relaxation.
- Dietitian – to maximize nutritional status and ensure adequate intake (particularly if therapeutic diets are attempted).
- Child psychiatrist – to aid diagnosis and identify depressive illness.
- Physiotherapist – to help devise a reasonable routine of exercise to aid recovery.
- Educationalist – to ensure school attendance and advise on alternative educational support if necessary.

Comments   Many other professionals may need to be involved in the approach to a child with such problems. The overall approach is to ensure some attendance at school and avoid social isolation. An increasing schedule of exercise and activities is necessary to promote recovery. The management of these cases remains very difficult.

The history provided is very variable and could potentially apply to many differing disorders. The symptoms commenced after a minor infection. Although he had been to the Mediterranean seaboard on holiday, there is no suggestion that he contracted a fever there. However, such infections must be considered. Mild holiday infections such as coliform diarrhoea is unlikely to last this long. Similarly, typhoid would be unusual in the absence of earlier symptoms. Brucellosis is one possibility, but unlikely. Leishmaniasis is excluded by the absence of hepatosplenomegaly. In view of the serology, an enteroviral aetiology is probable.

Chronic fatigue and all his other symptoms could represent infectious mononucleosis. Both the unreliable Monospot and specific serology are negative. Lymphoma or leukaemia are excluded by clinical findings and the blood film. Hypothyroidism is excluded on the basis of a normal TSH. Autoimmune serology is essentially normal, although a weakly positive anti-smooth muscle antibody titre was detected, which is most likely to be a nonspecific result of the preceding infection. An intracranial tumour is excluded by the normal MRI. There are no changes suggestive of a progressive neurodegenerative disorder or encephalitic process. SLE could potentially cause such problems, but a florid presentation would be less likely in the absence of further abnormal autoimmune serology. Poisoning should be considered in all cases where there seems to be unusual pathology.

In the absence of the above, his continued and varied symptomatology begins to suggest a major behavioural component. It is difficult to link all the symptoms under one diagnostic label. A multidisciplinary approach discovered family tensions associated with unresolved maternal feelings about her brother's death. The boy was quiet and admitted to worries about his mother. These had been exacerbated by his school examinations. The probable precipitating event was an enteroviral illness, which then caused chronic fatigue syndrome in a psychologically susceptible individual. Depressive illness remains a possibility.

Subsequent therapy by the psychologist in conjunction with the physiotherapist allowed a full recovery.

Answer 5.5

a) Paracentesis with biochemical analysis of ascites.
   Abdominal ultrasound with inferior vena cava (IVC) Doppler studies.
   Urinary albumin/creatinine ratio.
   24-hour urinary protein excretion.
   Renal ultrasound.
   Renal biopsy.
   Placental weight.
   IVC venography.

b) Congenital nephrotic syndrome.
   IVC thrombosis.

c) Denys–Drash syndrome (abnormal gonadal differentiation, nephropathy and nephroblastoma).

Comments   Although premature, the major feature of this infant is the oedema, which was massive. A central line had been *in situ* within the IVC. A thrombus may have formed resulting in occlusion. The renal function would resultantly fail with oedema, ascites and renal failure. The albumin is extremely low suggesting a congenital nephrotic syndrome.

Congenital nephrotic syndrome may be idiopathic, secondary, or associated with a syndrome. Idiopathic disease is often autosomal recessive in inheritance. Prematurity, placentomegaly, oedema and growth failure occur. Oedema occurs early, and although usually selective, becomes massive later. Renal failure occurs before the age of two years. Secondary causes are associated with infections such as syphilis and toxoplasmosis.

Several syndromes are associated with congenital nephrotic syndrome. The Denys–Drash syndrome is currently under investigation regarding antenatal markers. XY gonadal dysgenesis, nail–patella syndrome and an association with CNS deformity also occur.

Mesangial sclerosis, a feature of many variants of congenital nephrotic syndrome, may be detected on ultrasound scanning, allowing early neonatal diagnosis. Antenatal diagnosis is not yet available. However, elevated amniotic fluid α-fetoprotein levels occur, as in this case, but are non-specific as shown here.

Answer 5.6

a) Thyroid auto-antibody screen.
    Thyroid isotope scan.
    Thyroid ultrasound.

b) Autoimmune thyroiditis.

c) Eventual return to biochemical euthyroid status, but with a 5–10% cumulative risk of irreversible hypothyroidism.

Comments   The description suggests painless subacute autoimmune thyroiditis. Although the girl is clinically euthyroid, the thyroid function tests show T3 toxicosis. The autoimmune thyroid serology is extremely abnormal, with high titres of both antithyroglobulin and antimicrosomal autoantibodies. Eventual hypothyroidism is common.

Answer 5.7

a) Precocious puberty.

b) The patient demonstrates precocious puberty, which according to the Tanner stage is in an appropriate pattern (i.e. consonant). The bone age is advanced by 3.8 years. The GnRH test reveals an elevated baseline set of gonadotrophins. There is an exaggerated response to GnRH. This indicates a gonadotrophin-dependent cause of the precocious puberty.

c) Monthly injections of a GnRH analogue, to prevent hormone release. The start of treatment may cause a release of sex steroids. Their effects are blocked by the transient short-term use of cyproterone acetate.

Comments These results suggest gonadotrophin-dependent precocious puberty, which is the commonest type in females. The cause is
usually premature activation of the hypothalmic–pituitary axis. In boys,
it often represents intracranial disease.

Answer 5.8

a) Suprapubic aspirate of urine with microscopy and culture.

b) Acid/base balance.
   Blood cultures.
   Creatinine.
   Renal ultrasound.
   Other renal investigations, including micturating cystourethrogram
   and isotope study.

c) Hyponatraemic seizures manifesting as apnoeic episodes. The most
   likely underlying diagnosis is urinary tract infection.

Comments Hyponatraemia secondary to renal loss is a common
feature of neonatal urinary tract infection, particularly if a kidney is
obstructed. The evidence of an infection is supported by a raised CRP
estimation.

Answer 5.9

a) The maternal serological status is positive for hepatitis B. However,
   the infectivity status is low, as shown by the positive e antibody, but
   negative for the e antigen.

b) Vaccination against hepatitis B. Some authorities suggest additional
   administration of immunoglobulin, although others reserve this for
   those with high infectivity due to acute viral replication (i.e. HBeAg
   positive).

Comments If maternal serological status reveals HBsAg and eAg
positivity, approximately 90% of babies will become infected with the
majority becoming chronic carriers. Perinatal transmission is reduced if
the mother is eAb positive but eAg negative. Intrauterine transmission
is rare, with the majority of infections being acquired perinatally. Infectivity is denoted by eAg status. Immunoglobulin should be given within
12 hours to those at high risk. Vaccination should be given to all with
any combination of serological results.

5

Answer 5.10

a) Primary sclerosing cholangitis (PSC).
   Autoimmune chronic active hepatitis (CAH).

b) Endoscopic retrograde pancreatocholangiography (ERCP).
   Liver biopsy.

c) Immunosuppressants, including glucocorticosteroids and azathioprine.

Comments Hepatic and biliary pathology may occur in inflammatory bowel disease in children. In primary sclerosing cholangitis (PSC), the transaminases are greatly elevated together with IgG. Autoantibodies may be elevated particularly ANA and smooth muscle antibody. PSC may progress to biliary cirrhosis. CAH is also associated with a high titre of various autoantibodies. Although transaminases are usually elevated as in PSC, albumin levels are low, PT is prolonged early in the disease and hyperbilirubinaemia is common. Therefore, PSC is more likely in the above case, although CAH cannot be excluded purely on the data provided.

Answer 5.11

a) Pneumothorax.
   Blocked or displaced endotracheal tube.
   Unrecognized inadequate ventilation due to worsening lung disease.
   Asynchronous ventilation.
   Mechanical ventilator fault.

b) Suction of endotracheal tube.
   Reintubation.
   Urgent chest radiography.
   Transillumination of chest.

c) Increase in peak inspiratory pressure.
   Ensure synchronous ventilation.
   Combined increase in ventilator rate and FiO_2.

Answer 5.12

a) 24-hour oesophageal pH probe study.

b) Significant gastro-oesophageal reflux.

c) Combination of H2 antagonist (ranitidine) and prokinetic (cisapride).

Comments Gastro-oesophageal reflux is common and best diagnosed on 24-hour oesophageal pH monitoring. This study reveals a reflux index of 26% (i.e. severe reflux). This is best treated using the above medication. Omeprazole may be substituted for ranitidine in the presence of oesophagitis. If medical therapy fails, a surgical approach may be indicated. Simple cases may be managed with antacids and thickeners before pH monitoring. Severe cases or those of 'silent' reflux need a pH study. The former may also require oesophagoscopy to delineate oesophagitis.

Answer 5.13

a) Benign hyperphosphatasaemia of infancy.

b) None. Monitoring of biochemistry advised.

Comments　The results show an elevated alkaline phosphatase level, but no other disorder of liver function. The isoenzymes confirm that the elevation is due to a bone source. The other results suggest that the acute infection and inflammation has settled. Benign hyperphosphatasaemia of infancy usually follows a viral illness. The result is often unsuspected and commonly causes concern. The aetiology is believed to be due to activation of macrophage-derived bone-forming cells. Resolution is spontaneous.

Answer 5.14

a) Mycoplasma IgM.
　Paired atypical (mycoplasma) serology.
　Cold agglutinins.
　Cryoglobulins.

b) Mycoplasma infection.

c) Encephalitis.
　Guillain-Barré syndrome.
　Transverse myelitis.
　Haemolytic anaemia.
　Thrombocytopenia.
　Bullous myringitis.
　Myocarditis.
　Pericarditis.
　Erythema multiforme.

to complications of Mycoplasmal infection

Pneumonia

Comments　The association of respiratory symptoms and intolerance of the fingers to cold stimulus suggests cold agglutinins. The most likely cause is a Mycoplasma infection. This is supported by the other investigation results. Cryoglobulinaemia is less likely. Mycoplasma IgM is rather unreliable, hence many laboratories' preference for paired sera. Mycoplasma infection is common in childhood. Infections have been associated with many complications, some of which are listed above.

5

Answer 5.15

a) Maple syrup urine disease.

b) General supportive care.
   Dietary manipulation.

Comments The pattern of illness – exacerbation of symptoms on resumption of feeds, but recovery when receiving intravenous fluids, is suggestive of a metabolic disease. Hypoglycaemia and hypocalcaemia can be excluded as causes from the results. The characteristic pattern of amino acid excretion is diagnostic. Acidosis and neurological features occur more frequently than hypoglycaemia in this condition. A diet low in leucine, valine and isoleucine is necessary. The prognosis is good if the disorder is diagnosed early.

Answer 5.16

a) Coeliac disease.
   Cystic fibrosis.
   Giardiasis.
   Carbohydrate malabsorption – especially primary or secondary lactase deficiency.

   Alternatives may include:

   - Cow's milk protein intolerance.
   - Schwachman's syndrome (exocrine pancreatic failure with neutropenia).
   - Congenital chloridorrhoea.
   - Abetalipoproteinaemia.
   - Lymphangiectasia.

b) Coeliac disease serology (antigliadin, reticulin and endomysium antibodies).
   Jejunal biopsy – microscopy and biochemical function tests.
   Faecal reducing substances and chromatography.
   Faecal occult blood test.
   Faecal microscopy and culture.
   Blood film for acanthocytes (abetalipoproteinaemia) and lymphocyte count (low in lymphangiectasia).
   Chloride estimation (plasma, urine and stool).
   Serum immunoreactive trypsin (low in Schwachman's syndrome).
   Triglyceride and cholesterol levels.
   Protein electrophoresis.

Comments This child has an obviously distended abdomen associated with failure to thrive and the passage of loose pungent stools. This all suggests a malabsorption picture. This problem may be differentiated into: mucosal defects (coeliac disease), pancreatic disorders, metabolic disturbances and structural anomalies (lymphangiectasia).

The investigations largely depend upon other clinical features. Coeliac disease autoantibody serology may be useful to determine whether a child needs a jejunal biopsy. IgA variants of antiendomysial antibody are the most specific tests, but caution is necessary as false negatives do occur due to the association with IgA deficiency in coeliac disease. Subsequent resolution of the positive autoantibodies should occur in response to therapy.

Abetalipoproteinaemia is a defect in the production of apoprotein B by the gut. Defective synthesis of LDLs occurs. This is autosomal recessive and results in steatorrhoea. Cholesterol levels are low and many features are a result of a deficiency of fat-soluble vitamins.

Schwachman's syndrome is an abnormality of exocrine pancreatic function associated with neutropenia and skeletal dysplasia. Renal tubular disorders may occur. There is evidence that serum immunoreactive trypsin levels are low in this disease.

Answer 5.17

a) Arthrogryposis multiplex congenita.

b) Cranial ultrasound scan.
   Nerve conduction study.
   Creatine kinase estimation.
   EMG.
   Karyotype.
   Muscle biopsy.
   Congenital infection screen.

c) Variable. There is usually some physical handicap associated with the severe limb deformity. This is the determinant of future mobility. There is usually no intellectual impairment.

Comments Arthrogryposis multiplex congenita is a rare condition associated with severe physical deformity. Some cases are associated with an obvious aetiology, but many remain without a cause. Neuromuscular aetiologies need excluding and there is some evidence that some babies are affected by first trimester coxsackie or enteroviral infection.

Treatment is multidisciplinary and involves orthopaedic and physiotherapy support in addition to all the therapists encountered in the child
development centre.

Answer 5.18

a) Oesophageal atresia.

b) Aspiration of feeds or secretions.

c) Polyhydramnios.

Comments This chest radiograph shows a curled nasogastric tube
in the upper oesophagus. The diagnosis was made postnatally on this
film. The baby was not fed and was given intravenous fluids. A replogle
tube on continuous suction was inserted and the baby nursed 'head-up'.
Subsequent findings at surgery revealed an atresia with a distal tracheo-
oesophageal fistula. This is the most common variant (87%). A primary
anastomosis was possible. The antenatal history was complicated by
polyhydramnios.

Subsequently this infant suffered marked gastro-oesophageal reflux,
which is a recognized problem in this disorder along with the 'brassy'
cough.

Answer 5.19

a) Cardiomegaly.

b) Left ventricular hypertrophy.
Deep Q waves and inverted T waves in left chest leads.

c) Anomalous left coronary artery.

d) Congestive cardiac failure.

Comments This infant presented with failure to thrive and tachypnoea. The latter was due to congestive cardiac failure, which was supported by the apparent clinical hepatomegaly. Screaming attacks had
occurred, probably as a result of myocardial ischaemia. The ECG and
chest radiograph are highly suggestive of anomalous left coronary
artery arising from the pulmonary trunk. These children are at risk of
sudden death due to myocardial infarction. Echocardiography confirmed the diagnosis. Once the cardiac failure had been controlled, a
surgical repair was possible.

Answer 5.20

a) Plexiform neurofibroma in neurofibromatosis type 1.

b) Axillary and inguinal freckling.
   Café au lait patches.
   Lisch nodules (iris hamartomas).
   Sphenoid dysplasia.
   Pseudoarthrosis.
   Optic glioma.

c) Multidisciplinary including:
   Paediatrician.
   Geneticist.
   Ophthalmologist.
   Orthopaedic surgeon.
   Dermatologist.
   Educational psychologist.
   Teacher.
   Neurofibromatosis support worker.
   Regular multidisciplinary clinic to monitor:
   Growth.
   Head size (approximately 40% have macrocephaly).
   Scoliosis (spinal tumour).
   Blood pressure (renal artery stenosis).
   Visual acuity (optic tumour).
   Dermal problems.
   Learning problems.

Comments The incidence is approximately 1:3000 in the UK. A series of features are necessary for the diagnosis. Inheritance is autosomal dominant, although many are spontaneous mutations. The gene for type 1 is on chromosome 17. There are many complications, some of which are outlined above and necessitate a combined multidisciplinary approach.

Answer 5.21

a) Pneumomediastinum.

b) Supportive intensive care.

Comments Pneumomediastinum is a common radiological finding in sick infants who are ventilated. It is a form of air leak occurring as air tracks through the pulmonary interstitium. Radiological differentiation from a pneumopericardium can be difficult. The latter is often well circumscribed and may in extreme cases cause tamponade.

Pneumomediastinum can usually be differentiated as air can be seen tracking up into the neck on the radiograph. Most resolve spontaneously.

Answer 5.22

a) CT brain scan.

b) Right anterior porencephalic cyst with ventricular dilatation.

c) Probable severe periventricular haemorrhage during neonatal period.

Comments   Porencephalic cysts are often large and generally communicate with the ipsilateral lateral ventricle. They arise from liquefaction of a previous haemorrhage or area of venous infarct. They differ from periventricular leucomalacia, which results from ischaemic damage. Cystic degeneration occurs, which may result in cyst coalescence, but the cysts do not usually communicate with the ventricular system.

This cyst resulted from a Grade 4 periventricular haemorrhage associated with a tension pneumothorax.

Answer 5.23

a) Cutis aplasia.

b) Patau's syndrome.
Idiopathic.
Other chromomosomal anomalies.

c) Karyotype.
Cranial ultrasound scan.
Skull radiograph.

Comments   Cutis aplasia (where the scalp is deficient) is a frequent association with trisomy 13 Patau's syndrome. It may be idiopathic or be confused with damage caused by a fetal scalp electrode. Other chromosomal defects have been associated with this problem. Usually no treatment is necessary as the smaller lesions granulate over spontaneously. Larger defects may need plastic surgery.

Answer 5.24

a) Thyroid goitre.

b) Thyroid function tests.
Thyroid autoantibody screen.
Thyroid isotope scan.
Bone age.

Comments A goitre is shown in this picture. The most common are euthyroid goitres and are usually due to thyroiditis. Thyroid function tests will identify the biochemical thyroid status. The autoimmune origin is often shown by the high titres of antithyroid autoantibodies, and this may be confirmed by thyroid isotope studies. In view of the risk of subsequent hypothyroidism, a baseline bone age estimation is of use for further assessment should thyroid or growth failure ensue.

Answer 5.25

a) Posterior mediastinal mass.

b) Thoracic neuroblastoma.

c) Urinary catecholamine/creatinine ratio. ✓
   Plasma catecholamines. ✓
   CT thorax scan. ✓
   Methyliodobenzylguanidine (MIBG) scan. ✓
   Biopsy of mass. ✓
   Adrenal and abdominal ultrasound or CT scan. ✓
   Bone marrow aspiration. ✓

d) Good prognosis.

Comments Neuroblastoma remains the most common extracranial solid tumour. Affected infants below one year of age have an improved prognosis compared with older children, particularly if associated with Stage 4S tumour (localized primary tumour with dissemination limited to liver, skin and/or bone marrow). Thoracic primaries occur in about 14% of cases. 60% arise from the abdomen. Cervical neuroblastoma may present with Horner's syndrome.

Diagnosis depends upon an elevated urinary catecholamine/creatinine ratio and positive biopsy or bone marrow aspirate. Immunohistochemistry and cytogenetics may aid diagnosis. Staging necessitates some of the following: CT or MRI of chest and abdomen; bone marrow aspiration; MIBG scan; ^{99}Tc diphosphonate bone scan if the MIBG scan is normal. At least 90% of neuroblastomas take up MIBG on scan.

This chest radiograph is from a child with Stage 2 disease, which has a high cure rate following surgery. Thoracic neuroblastomas are usually more differentiated than abdominal tumours of identical stage and therefore have a better prognosis.

Answer 5.26

a) Psoriasis.

b) Topical glucocorticosteroids.
   Tar-based preparations.
   Dithranol.

Comments   Psoriasis may be variable in presentation, colour and distribution. Younger infants may suffer with lesions in the nappy area. Winter accentuation is common. Pustular psoriasis is a severe form. Both photochemotherapy and potent oral corticosteroids are contraindicated in children.

Answer 5.27

a) Meconium aspiration syndrome.

b) Combination of atelectasis and alveolar collapse and pneumonitis. The former results in ventilation–perfusion mismatch. The pneumonitis may cause pulmonary oedema. The result is often severe pulmonary hypertension with intrapulmonary shunting. Secondary infection often intervenes. Studies indicate that meconium may inactivate endogenous surfactant.

c) Maximize oxygenation.
   Maximize ventilation including mechanical ventilation.
   Prevent pulmonary hypertension or treat if present.
   General intensive care.
   Antibiotic therapy.
   Consider surfactant administration, nitric oxide inhaled therapy if refractory hypoxia occurs, extracorporeal membrane oxygenation (ECMO).

Comments   Meconium aspiration can cause severe respiratory failure associated with refractory hypoxia. Prevention is important, although undoubtedly some infants will aspirate before delivery during the second stage of labour. Surfactant therapy may be beneficial. These babies may be extremely difficult to ventilate and may suffer airleaks. Severely ill babies with pulmonary hypertension may benefit from nitric oxide therapy or need ECMO.

Answer 5.28

a) Herpes zoster (shingles).

b) Hospital admission.
   Intravenous acyclovir.

Comments This infant is immunocompromised (considered to be so for at least six months following cessation of chemotherapy). There is a risk of severe disseminated varicella. Therefore intravenous therapy is necessary bearing in mind the limited oral bioavailability of acyclovir. Intravenous therapy is continued until there are no new lesions, then oral acyclovir is used until the lesions have healed. New drugs like famciclovir may be more orally bioavailable and may alter the above approach when further experience is available.

Answer 5.29

a) Alopecia associated with Down's syndrome.

b) Intellectual impairment.
   Slow growth.
   Effects of cardiac or gastrointestinal malformation.
   Constipation.
   Hyperkeratosis.
   Cataracts.
   Visual defects.
   Sleep apnoea.
   Increased susceptibility to infection.
   Leukaemia.
   Seizures.
   Hypothyroidism and other autoimmune diseases.

Answer 5.30

a) Coloured urine suggestive of a conjugated prolonged hyperbilirubinaemia.

Prolonged Jaundice screen

b) Bilirubin – conjugated and total.
   Liver function tests.
   PT.
   Liver and biliary ultrasound scan.
   Serial stool collections monitoring degree of cholestasis.
   Congenital infection serology and urinary isolation.
   α-1-antitrypsin phenotype.
   Urinary reducing substances for galactosaemia.
   Amino acids – plasma and urinary.
   Organic acids – urinary.
   DISIDA (HIDA) isotope excretion liver scan.
   Others – bone marrow aspirate, liver biopsy.   → *Thyroid Function Tests.*

5

c) Pale yellow–white.

Comments   This infant has prolonged (greater than 14 days) neonatal jaundice. The presence of highly coloured urine is suggestive of a conjugated type, which would be supported by cholestatic stools and confirmed by analysis of the fractions of serum bilirubin.

Conjugated hyperbilirubinaemia is uncommon in the neonatal period. Its importance lies in the need to diagnose surgically remediable anomalies (e.g. biliary atresia) early to allow surgery. The best results following surgery for extrahepatic biliary atresia are seen when surgery occurs before 60 days of life. After this time, portal hypertension ensues and the likelihood of bile flow is drastically reduced. Similarly, abnormalities that may be amenable to dietary manipulation will benefit from early diagnosis. The major possible diagnoses include:

● Biliary atresia and other surgical problems.
● Congenital infection.
● Total parenteral nutrition.
● Idiopathic hepatitis.
● α-1-antitrypsin deficiency, particularly PiZZ.
● Galactosaemia.
● Tyrosinaemia.
● Other metabolic disorders.
● Endocrine abnormalities (e.g. septo-optic dysplasia, panhypopituitarism).

Answer 5.31

a) Generalized osteopenic appearance.
   Splaying of the metaphyses.
   Ragged appearance of the metaphyseal plate.
   Bowing of the legs.

b) Rickets – probably nutritional.

c) Appropriate dietary advice.
   Vitamin D supplementation.

Comments   The radiography shows the characteristic appearance of rickets. Clinically this child is short, bowlegged, weak with a proximal myopathy, expanded wrists and persisting anterior fontanelle. The aetiology is vitamin D deficiency resulting from the sole use of breast milk and failure to wean. Subsequent treatment with vitamin D resulted in complete resolution of the physical abnormalities while allowing attainment of the expected milestones. In boys without such a predisposing history, hypophosphataemic rickets must also be considered.

Answer 5.32

a) Goldenhar's syndrome.

b) Cleft palate.
Cardiac defects.
Ocular abnormalities.
Skeletal, particularly vertebral, anomalies.
Developmental delay.

Comments   Goldenhar's syndrome has a variable autosomal inheritance with widely disparate incidences of 1:5600 to 1:26000. There is a slight male predominance. Characteristic features include:

- Abnormalities of pinna and middle ear.
- Hemifacial asymmetry.
- Micrognathia and feeding problems.
- Cleft palate, occasionally with a cleft lip.
- Colobomas.
- Narrow palpebral fissures.
- Scoliosis and hemivertebrae with bifid ribs.
- Cardiac defects, particularly VSDs. *ToP*
- Dental problems.
- Emotional and intellectual problems.

Alternative titles include ocular-auriculo-vertebral anomaly and first and second branchial arch syndrome.

Answer 5.33

a) Lichenified eczema.

b) Emollients.
Topical glucocorticosteroid.

Comments   Lichenification is a feature of chronic eczema. It is scaly, dry and often pruritic.

Answer 5.34

a) Congenital hydrocephalus.

b) Full wide anterior fontanelle.
'Sunsetting' eyes.
Distended scalp vessels.
Cracked pot sign on percussion.
Parting of the sutures.
Occasionally papilloedema, optic atrophy, irritability.

c) Arnold–Chiari malformation.
   Congenital associated with syndromes (Dandy–Walker).
   Congenital infection (particularly toxoplasmosis).
   Idiopathic.
   Aqueduct stenosis (nonsyndromic and syndromic – X-linked with adducted thumbs).
   CSF overproduction – choroid plexus papilloma.
   Postneonatal meningitis.
   Posterior fossa arachnoid cyst.
   Aneurysmal dilatation of the vein of Galen.
   In the preterm infant: Post haemorrhage (not in this case).

Comments This CT brain scan shows marked hydrocephalus without obvious cause. There is asymptomatic calcification in one choroid plexus. If treatment is necessary then ventriculoperitoneal shunting is usually the standard therapy. In the preterm infant, trials continue where CSF production is reduced using a carbonic anhydrase inhibitor (acetazolamide) and frusemide.

Answer 5.35

a) Gianotti Crosti syndrome.

b) Hepatitis B.
   Mycoplasma spp.
   Coxsackie A and B.
   EBV.

Comments Infantile papular acrodermatitis (Gianotti Crosti syndrome) was originally described in association with hepatitis B infection although several other infections have now been implicated. The rash is predominantly over the face and peripheries avoiding the trunk. The erythema may become purpuric in areas. Liver function tests usually reveal elevated transaminase levels. Treatment is symptomatic.

EXAM
ANSWERS

1

2

3

4

5

6

ANSWERS - Exam 6
Answer 6.1

a) Peripheral neuropathy secondary to trauma-induced arteriovenous malformation or traumatic false aneurysm.

b) Doppler ultrasound.
   MRI angiography.

Comments   The initial symptoms suggest a neuropathy. A variety of causes are possible from the history including trauma, Guillain–Barré syndrome, poliomyelitis, toxic neuropathy, metabolic neuropathy, migraine, intracranial tumour, multiple sclerosis and psychogenic causes.

Examination reveals a demarcated sensory neuropathy. The absence of motor dysfunction excludes Guillain–Barré syndrome and poliomyelitis. There is no evidence of progression of signs or prodromal illness of myalgia, both of which would be more characteristic of these alternative diagnoses. Toxic neuropathies rarely present acutely, even following diphtheria. Similarly there are no features of a metabolic disturbance in the history, particularly a disorder such as acute intermittent porphyria. There is no significant family history.

Jenny's headaches were not progressive and had yielded to simple analgesia, thus making the possibility of an intracranial mass unlikely. A psychogenic cause cannot be excluded on the above history, but there is no obvious reason for Jenny to have psychogenic headaches, particularly as they had resolved after changing schools. There are insufficient features to diagnose the rare juvenile multiple sclerosis. Furthermore there is no imaging or biochemical supporting evidence.

The symptoms seem to be temporally related to trauma. Spinal injury is excluded by imaging. However, the nerve conduction studies are abnormal, indicating sural nerve pressure. Although standard ultrasonography is normal, there is a suggestion of an ill-defined buttock mass, which could be impinging on the sensory nerve supply. A soft bruit indicates abnormal blood flow in the buttock. Therefore, in view of the history, the most likely aetiology is trauma giving rise to abnormal vascular flow. Indeed, further investigations revealed a traumatic false aneurysm pressing on the sensory nerves in the buttock. This was identified using MRI angiography.

6

Answer 6.2

a) Tuberous sclerosis.

b) Cardiac rhabdomyoma.

c) Facial angiofibromas (adenoma sebaceum).
   Periungual fibromas.
   Calcified retinal hamartomas.
   Cortical tubers.
   Subependymal glial nodules.
   Bilateral renal angiomyolipomas.
   Forehead fibrous plaque.
   Shagreen patch.
   Hypomelanic macules.
   Bilateral polycystic kidneys.
   Radiographic honeycomb lung.

Comments   The presenting complaint is a prolonged seizure associated with fever. At seven years of age this boy is out of the typical age range for febrile convulsions and the length of the seizure is quite prolonged for this diagnosis. Meningitis is a real possibility. This is not excluded by the absence of fever on admission, but this reduces its likelihood. The elevated WCC may be due to fever or post-seizure. However, all cultures and infection markers are normal.

There is a history of minor head trauma. Trauma cannot therefore be excluded although the timing is rather too long except for a slow extradural haemorrhage as a cause. Significant damage is unlikely as there is no history of loss of consciousness after the accident. Similarly there is no obvious fracture. The CT scan does not reveal intracranial damage.

Other possible diagnoses include sickle neurological crisis (but the Hb electrophoresis is normal) and the possibility of drug ingestion and poisoning. The electrolyte pattern is not helpful as the hyponatraemia and hyperglycaemia probably result from the prolonged seizure. The presence of a heart murmur might indicate an embolic phenomenon or the presence of a subsequent abscess. There are no features of the former and the latter should be associated with a spiking fever and focal neurological signs. The neurological signs described are caused by the ictal state of this boy.

The association of the seizure, skin stigmas and learning disability is suggestive of tuberous sclerosis. This is confirmed by the typical CT appearance. This appearance occurs in 85% of patients. Once the diagnosis is confirmed additional features can be sought, including the real reason for the heart murmur. The echocardiogram revealed not a VSD, but cardiac tumour. These are the earliest hamartomas in this disorder. They occur in over 50% of children with this disorder and may even be identified antenatally from 22 weeks' gestation. Most are asymptomatic, but others can cause cardiac failure, arrthymias or murmurs.

Answer 6.3

a) Sweat test.
   Cystic fibrosis gene probe.
   Oesophagoscopy.
   Contrast oesophagram.
   Barium swallow.
   Immune studies.
   Ciliary studies.

b) Cystic fibrosis.

c) Physiotherapy.
   Prophylactic flucloxacillin during first year of life.
   Pancreatic supplements.
   Vitamins, particularly A, D, E and K.
   Bronchodilators if necessary.
   Calorific supplementation if necessary.
   Prevention of infection.

Comments   The scenario poses the problem of a severe non-RSV atypical bronchiolitis. The baby does not seem to recover in the usual manner, so an underlying problem must be considered. The underlying possibilities include immunodeficiency, pulmonary disease, cardiac disease and upper gastrointestinal problems with or without aspiration.

From the history, there is no evidence of chronic lung disease and no significant neonatal problems. However, the 'bronchiolitic' illness may be the presenting feature of a chronic illness. The changing radiographic appearance may be part of the same disorder (e.g. mucous plugging of the airway) or a secondary phenomenon (e.g. bacterial infection). There is documented poor weight gain and a convalescent oxygen dependency. This is unusual for typical bronchiolitis and raises the possibility of a systemic disorder such as cystic fibrosis. Each year cases of cystic fibrosis are revealed following severe or prolonged respiratory symptoms associated with bronchiolitis.

Gastro-oesophageal reflux is common and may account for wheezing and coughing in those with and without respiratory disease. The situation is exacerbated if aspiration occurs. Vomiting is a poor indicator

6

of reflux although there may be a history of being 'sicky'. However, the reflux index is normal. As this measures acid reflux, total reflux, including milk, may be underrepresented. An H-type tracheo-oesophageal fistula could present in a similar manner with recurrent aspiration. Diagnosis is difficult and may require a combination of oesophagoscopy and radiographic measures. There is no evidence of a cardiac lesion. Immune studies to exclude generalized deficiency need consideration.

The most likely diagnosis resulting from the combination of chronic respiratory problems, complicated bronchiolitis and poor weight gain since birth remains cystic fibrosis. Management centres upon a multi-system approach with attention to growth, chest physiotherapy, early treatment of acute infections, prophylactic antistaphylococcal antibiotics, pancreatic supplementation and adequate vitamin replacement.

Answer 6.4

a) Haemolytic uraemic syndrome (HUS).

b) Blood film showing red cell fragments and burr cells.
   Evidence of *Escherichia coli* 0157 in stools.

c) Beefburger.

d) General supportive care.
   Fresh frozen plasma.
   Renal support, including dialysis if necessary.

Comments   The key feature of this case is the association of thrombocytopenic purpura, seizure and bloody diarrhoea. There is a short period of time between the diarrhoea and the convulsion. The blood investigations reveal an elevated WCC which could be due to the seizure. There is anaemia together with the thrombocytopenia. Hyponatraemia is associated with renal impairment, including haematuria and proteinuria. There is a slightly elevated bilirubin level.

The differential diagnosis includes meningococcaemia with or without meningitis. This should always be considered in the scenario of seizure and thrombocytopenic purpura in an ill child. There is no clear evidence that there is a meningococcal infection from the results given. Idiopathic thrombocytopenic purpura may occur after a trivial infection, but is rarely accompanied by such ill health or renal dysfunction. Severe dehydration is clinically and biochemically unlikely as a diagnosis and does not fit in with the time course of the illness. If surgical causes of bloody diarrhoea are considered, inflammatory bowel disease is rare below 8–10 years of age. Intussusception is a possibility, although seizures only occur secondary to severe electrolyte disturbance. The pattern of the disease progression is unlikely for this diagnosis.

Infective gastroenteritis remains the most likely problem. Most bacterial enterides can cause bloody diarrhoea with Campylobacter being the most common. However, shigellae are the most likely to cause severe neurological complications sufficient to mimic meningitis. Therefore shigellae are a possible aetiological group. Salmonellae and clostridia are also possible causes.

The renal dysfunction has arisen after the acute illness and seems unrelated to dehydration. The association of anaemia and hyperbilirubinaemia suggests a haemolytic component. The combination of all these makes the diagnosis of HUS likely. This is usually a result of infection with verocytotoxin-producing *E. coli* 0157, which causes a microangiopathic haemolytic anaemia with renal dysfunction.

HUS is often associated with a preceding illness characterized by bloody diarrhoea. There may be clusters of infection which predominate in the spring and summer months. It is usually seen in children under 5 years of age. Treatment is largely supportive, although HUS is one of the most common causes of acute renal failure in the paediatric age group. The mortality is 2–10%.

Answer 6.5

a) TPN pleural collection.
   Pleural effusions or chylothorax.
   Worsening lung pathology including infection.
   Inadequate ventilation.
   Cardiac failure due to a patent ductus arteriosus.
   Pneumothorax.

b) Chest radiograph, including administration of radio-opaque dye to outline the silastic long line.
   Chest ultrasound scan.
   Echocardiogram.
   Biochemical analysis of secretions.
   Microbiological analysis of secretions.

c) TPN pleural collection.

d) Thoracocentesis and analysis of the fluid.

e) Post-insertion identification, with dye, of the position of the line.
   Secure fixing of the line to prevent intravascular migration.

6

Comments   There is a progressive deterioration in respiratory function, which may be endogenous (i.e. worsening of the lung pathology or pleural effusion) or exogenous (i.e. misplaced endotracheal tube). Any problem with the endotracheal tube was checked by reintubation. This would be the most likely problem if there had been a sudden deterioration in this infant's clinical state.

If the collapse had been sudden, a pneumothorax is a likely possibility. Although a gradual deterioration does not exclude this diagnosis, the time course plus the absence of chest transillumination and the patient-triggered mode of ventilation make this less likely.

Infection may cause a deterioration. Although there is a history of group B streptococcal carriage, the mother was treated during delivery with ampicillin, which is known to reduce the risk of infection. A nosocomial infection is a possibility, although the baby is only three days old. The CRP concentration does not support a bacterial infection.

An intracranial haemorrhage could potentially cause such a decline, although massive bleeding usually accompanies some other neonatal complication particularly sepsis or coagulopathy and occurs within 72 hours of delivery. The copious secretions could result from inflammation or be part of the intravenous feed. The chest radiograph reveals a suddenly-occurring unilateral abnormality. This is on the side of the silastic long line. A chest ultrasound showed a pleural collection, which was shown to be TPN on analysis after thoracocentesis. Further radiological studies showed that the long line was positioned in the right-sided pulmonary vasculature and that TPN had passed into the lung interstitium and then into the pleural space and airway. Subsequent repositioning of the line and thoracocentesis cured the problem with eventual resolution of the respiratory and radiographic signs.

Answer 6.6

a) Haemophilia A.

b) Investigation to identify the degree of production of factor VIII in response to a pharmacological dose of desmopressin.

c) In view of the poor response to desmopressin, this child's ENT operation requires perioperative administration of exogenous factor VIII cryoprecipitate.

Comments   The coagulation tests show a prolonged APTT but normal thrombin time and PT. The interpretation of this is a deficiency of factors VIII, IX, XI or XII. The individual factor VIII assays indicate a deficiency of the coagulant, but not related antigen. This makes Von Willebrand's disease unlikely and haemophilia A more likely. The RiCOF or Von Willebrand's factor (VWF) is normal, therefore confirming the above. Although some people with haemophilia A will mount a good response to DDAVP, this must be proven before undertaking a potentially hazardous surgical procedure. Ideally the VIIIc level should be maintained above 0.5 and preferably at 0.8–1.0 preoperatively.

Answer 6.7

a) Congenital adrenal hypoplasia.

b) Short synacthen test.
Urinary steroid profile.

c) Glycerol kinase deficiency.
Myopathy.
Gonadotrophin deficiency.
Deafness.

Comments The electrolyte pattern suggests salt loss and both dehydration and hypoglycaemia. An adrenal aetiology is supported by the elevated ACTH result. Congenital adrenal hyperplasia (CAH) due to 21-hydroxylase deficiency, the most common defect, is excluded by the normal 17-hydroxyprogesterone level. As the child is male (no sexual ambiguity is mentioned in the question) the only cases of CAH with a normal 17-hydroxyprogesterone (17-hydroxylase deficiency and lipoid adrenal hyperplasia) are excluded as these cause male sexual ambiguity. Therefore congenital adrenal hypoplasia is the most likely diagnosis. This may be diagnosed by the failure to produce cortisol following a short synacthen test and the absence of gonadotrophins. Although classically X-linked, some cases are sporadic or autosomal recessive.

Answer 6.8

a) Drug withdrawal.
Hyponatraemia.
Cerebral malformation.

b) Opiate withdrawal can result in seizures that only respond to opiate administration. This is a biochemical effect upon endorphin receptors.

Hyponatraemia can result from inappropriate vasopressin secretion stimulated by maternal polydrug abuse via uncertain mechanisms. The low osmolality may be indicative of this situation.

6

Cerebral malformations may occur following an embryopathy associated with early pregnancy drug abuse.

Comments   Cocaine may cause cerebral infarction due to its vasoactive function. All babies born to those abusing cocaine should have a cranial ultrasound scan.

Answer 6.9

a) Supraventricular tachycardia (SVT) on ECG.

b) Adenosine bolus intravenously 0.05–0.25 mg/kg.

Comments   This ECG shows an SVT resulting from an atrioventricular (AV) re-entry accessory pathway or nodal phenomenon. Adenosine is the drug of choice. It blocks conduction through the AV node. Usually non-pharmacological therapies (i.e. vagal stimulation) will be attempted with varying degrees of success. Flushing, anxiety and chest tightness are all transient side-effects. Other therapies include digoxin, flecainide, propranolol, verapamil and synchronized DC shock.

Answer 6.10

a) Hereditary angio-oedema.

b) Fresh frozen plasma.
   Hydrocortisone.

c) Usually autosomal dominant.

Comments   The investigations show a functional deficiency of C1 inhibitor. Acquired aetiology occurs but this is usually in adults with SLE or proliferative malignancy where the disorder is characterized by low C1q levels. All types are associated, as in this case, with a low C4. Chronic treatment is with danazol (increases production) and tranexamic acid (reduces consumption).

Answer 6.11

a) Blood glucose level.
   Paracetamol level.
   Salicylate level.
   Electrolyte assay.
   Urinary toxicology.
   PT.

b) Salicylate (aspirin).

c) General supportive care.
   Maintenance of airway.

Gastric lavage after intubation.
Activated charcoal after lavage.
Intravenous dextrose saline.
Intravenous bicarbonate.
Consider acetazolamide, vitamin K, alkaline diuresis, dialysis.
ALWAYS CONTACT THE NEAREST POISONS UNIT FOR
UP-TO-DATE ADVICE.

Comments The blood gas result shows a partially compensated
metabolic acidosis with hypocarbia. This is most likely to be due to
aspirin poisoning. In this situation, initial hyperventilation produces a
respiratory alkalosis with base loss in the urine to compensate. Subsequently a metabolic acidosis occurs. Carbohydrate metabolic dysfunction results in hypoglycaemia and ketosis. Dehydration and
hypoprothrombinaemia also occur.

Answer 6.12

a) Early puberty: G2–3, P2–3, A0–1.

b) Constitutional delay in growth and puberty (CDGP).

c) Observation.
   Anabolic androgens: oxandrolone.
   Testosterone derivatives: oral or intramuscular.

Comments The growth chart shows a boy with growth failure with a
probable onset at around ten years of age. His growth had slowed
considerably although there is evidence that he is now starting to grow
after his fifteenth birthday. The most likely diagnosis is CDGP, which is
the association of growth delay and pubertal delay. It is much more
common in males. At this stage in his growth, he is probably in early puberty, which is reflected in his Tanner staging. The most likely testicular
volumes using an orchidometer are 4–8 ml. If no treatment is instituted,
he will eventually undergo a late growth spurt with pubertal development, although this can be accelerated by using the above medications.

Answer 6.13

a) Henoch–Schönlein purpura (HSP).

b) Immune complex-mediated type III hypersensitivity reaction

c) Renal involvement (rarely renal failure – usually haematuria and
   proteinuria).
   Intussusception.
   Generalized abdominal pain.
   Gastrointestinal haemorrhage.

6

Arthritis.
Nervous system involvement.
Scrotal pain and testicular swelling.

Comments This case is one of non-thrombocytopenic purpura. The clotting profile is normal. Immune complexes are present and there is an elevated serum IgA level Therefore HSP is the most likely diagnosis. Abnormal clotting or thrombocytopenia should be present in a bleeding diathesis or acute meningococcaemia.

Answer 6.14

a) Hyperinsulinism.

b) Insulin level. ✓
   C peptide level. ✓

c) Hydrocortisone.
   Diazoxide with chlorothiazide.
   Somatostatin infusion.
   Subtotal pancreatectomy.

Comments The current glucose requirements are 16.3 mg glucose/ kg/minute. (i.e. mg glucose/kg/minute = $(10 \times \%\text{dextrose} \times \text{ml/h})/$ (weight (kg) $\times$ 60)). Values above 12 are highly suggestive of hyperinsulinism. Even this delivery rate is insufficient as this baby is still hypoglycaemic (1.8 mmol/l). Hyperinsulinism may be associated with maternal diabetes mellitus, Beckwith syndrome, nesidioblastosis and ß-cell adenoma. Rarely it may accompany severe rhesus haemolytic disease.

Answer 6.15

a) Normal water deprivation test.

b) Habit.
   Probably associated with persistent mouth breathing associated with adenoidal hypertrophy.

Comments The water deprivation test reveals a normal concentrating ability. Although the urinary osmolality does not quite reach 800 mOsm/kg, this is the most likely a result of his large oral intake of fluids. This is, in turn, probably a result of mouth breathing due to his large adenoid, which has been removed. During the test there was no significant weight loss nor a major increase in plasma osmolality.

Answer 6.16

a) Bilateral perihilar shadowing in the middle and lower lobes.

b) Atypical pneumonia (Mycoplasma).

c) Paired sera for Mycoplasma.
   Mycoplasma IgM.
   Cold agglutinins.

d) Haemolytic anaemia.
   Thrombocytopenia.
   Arthralgia.
   Meningoencephalitis.
   Guillain–Barré syndrome.
   Transverse myelitis.

Comments This chest radiograph has bilateral abnormalities without a lobar distribution making an atypical aetiology or possibly bronchopneumonia likely. The absence of signs suggests an atypical aetiology. The association with haemolysis and rouleaux suggests that Mycoplasma is the causative organism. Initially considered a pneumonia of adults and adolescents, Mycoplasma is frequently seen in children, but only rarely in babies.

Answer 6.17

a) Right lung hyperexpansion.
   Segmental collapse in the left lingular and lower lobes.

b) Bilateral foreign body.

c) Partial obstruction in the right main bronchus acting as a 'ball valve' and complete obstruction in a divisional left bronchus causing complete collapse of the distal lung.

Comments Although the right main bronchus remains the favoured site of inhaled foreign bodies, both the trachea and the left bronchi may be affected. In this case, the skin and fragment of a peanut were recovered from the right side and a whole peanut from the left.

Answer 6.18

a) Erythema multiforme.

b) Drugs (e.g. antibiotics and non-steroidal anti-inflammatory medication).
   Streptococcal disease.
   Mycoplasma infection.

6

Infectious mononucleosis.
Autoimmune disease (e.g. SLE).

c) Symptomatic only.

Comments Erythema multiforme is usually a dermatological manifestation of systemic illness or drug therapy. Stevens–Johnson syndrome
is much more severe with mucosal involvement and often requires
systemic glucocorticosteroid therapy.

Answer 6.19

a) Intravenous urogram (IVU).

b) Malrotated right kidney with partial pelviureteric junction obstruction.

c) The obstruction only becomes clinically significant when there is a
urinary diuresis, such as after drinking alcohol.

Comments The IVU shows an unusual pattern of calyces, which
suggests malrotation. A previous scan, when asymptomatic, did not
reveal obstruction. However this IVU, taken during pain, shows the
partial obstruction. In this case, the degree of obstruction was mild. It
arose from an overlying aberrant blood vessel, which only obstructed
the pelvis significantly when the pelvis dilated during a diuresis – a complication of lager drinking!

Answer 6.20

a) Craniosynostosis.

b) Premature fusion of the metopic (forehead frontal) suture.

c) Surgical if there is evidence of raised intracranial pressure, ophthal-
mic complications or cosmetic concerns.

Comments This is a relatively unusual type of craniosynostosis with
isolated fusion of the metopic suture. Corresponding increased growth
in the other planes gives rise to the overall appearance. It is usually more
of cosmetic than of neurosurgical concern.

Answer 6.21

a) Massive right parietal intracranial haemorrhage.

b) Vascular malformation.

Comments This acute CT scan shows a massive intracranial haemorrhage, which was sadly fatal. There is evidence of intracranial com-

pression due to a mass effect. At autopsy, a vascular malformation was noted. It is conceivable that the preceding illness associated with protracted vomiting may have predisposed to vessel rupture.

Answer 6.22

a) Scalp candidiasis.

b) Topical and, if necessary, systemic antifungal therapy.

Comments This girl had other sites of recurrent candidiasis. She has mucocutaneous candidiasis. Further investigations revealed abnormal autoimmune serology with positive serology against the thyroid and adrenal glands.

Answer 6.23

a) Thymic shadow.

b) Not necessary! If uncertain, CT thoracic scans or fluoroscopy may occasionally be helpful. ECG to exclude cardiomegaly is rarely necessary.

Comments The thymic shadow is a common finding on the infantile chest radiograph. It may drape itself over either side of the heart border or sit centrally as in this case. The unwary may be concerned about the possibility of cardiomegaly or heart failure. The other classic appearance is the sail sign where there is a sharp demarcated lower border of the thymus on the right side of the chest mimicking an upper lobe consolidation.

Answer 6.24

a) Micturating cystourethrogram (MCUG).

b) Bilaterally massively dilated ureters with bilateral hydronephrosis due to massive bilateral vesicoureteric reflux.

c) Antibiotic prophylaxis.
   Radioisotope scan (DMSA) to identify renal insufficiency and scarring.
   Bilateral ureteric reimplantation is likely to be necessary.

Comments This MCUG reveals both hydroureters and hydronephrosis. This appearance could be due to posterior urethral valves, although there is no evidence of this on this particular scan. If not then severe reflux is most likely. With this severity, renal function is likely to deteriorate so ureteric reimplanation will probably be necessary.

6

Answer 6.25

a) Increased skin pigmentation over her fingers with evidence of vene-
section.

b) Addison's disease.

c) Serial cortisol assays.
Short synacthen test.
ACTH level.
Electrolytes.
Urinary electrolyte levels.
Autoantibody screen.

d) Both glucocorticoidsteroid and mineralocortico replacement.

Comments   This girl suffered a hypoglycaemic seizure. Hypoadrenalism is one cause of such a seizure and is supported by the increased
pigmentation shown. The diagnosis is made on the basis of an absent
response to synacthen. Acutely, cortisol levels may be low in addition to
the elevated ACTH and possible electrolyte disturbance. Most cases of
Addison's disease are autoimmune in nature with positive serology. Dual
replacement is necessary. Monitoring response to the glucocorticosteroid
is by serial ACTH assessment. Mineralocorticoid function is difficult
to monitor, but this may be achieved using plasma renin activity and
serum potassium levels.

Answer 6.26

a) Small bowel obstruction.

b) Analgesia.
Nasogastric tube insertion and suction.
Intravenous fluids.
General supportive care.
Surgical referral.

Comments   This radiograph shows extremely dilated loops of small
bowel. This is consistent with profuse bilious vomiting and suggests
obstruction. In this case, the obstruction was due to a malrotation with
obstruction by Ladd's bands.

Answer 6.27

a) Constipation.

b) Combination of:

● Increased fluid intake.
● Appropriate diet.

- Stool softener.
- Bowel stimulant (senna) when stools are soft.
- Assessment of psychological or behavioural factors.
- Rarely suppository or enema.

Comments Faecal loading is often seen on radiography. This is a severe picture of constipation. Abdominal radiographs are not routinely necessary for constipation although they can sometimes be used to help plan management or aid explanation to the parents and child.

Answer 6.28

a) Right inguinal hernia – gas-filled loops of bowel appearing in the pelviscrotal area on radiography.

b) The preterm infant is more at risk of inguinal hernias due to prematurity and (usually) mechanical ventilation.

Comments Inguinal hernias are very common in preterm infants. They have a high risk of incarceration and subsequent strangulation. A herniotomy is advised as a priority to prevent this complication, which has a significant morbidity in this group of infants.

Answer 6.29

a) Cardiomegaly.
   Pulmonary oedema.
   Pleural effusions.

b) First degree heart block.

c) Rheumatic fever.

d) Arthritis.
   Nodules.
   Chorea.
   Erythema marginatum.
   Minor criteria: elevated acute phase reactants; elevated WCC; fever; arthralgia; raised ASOT titre.

e) Aspirin or other nonsteroidal anti-inflammatory drugs.
   Glucocorticosteroids for carditis.
   Penicillin.

Comments Rheumatic fever is rare in the UK. The diagnosis is made by fulfilling the modified Jones criteria. Acute carditis may occur associated with or without first degree heart block. The treatment remains controversial although glucocorticosteroid therapy may be life saving.

6

Answer 6.30

a) Hydrocephalous.

b) Ventriculoperitoneal shunting.

c) Pineal tumour.

Comments   The association of headaches and progressive neurological deficit is an indication for further investigation. This MRI scan shows hydrocephalous. There is a defined pineal tumour, which is believed to be the underlying cause of the obstructive hydrocephalous. This is a slow growing tumour. Growth of the mass prompted surgical resection.

Answer 6.31

a) Acute respiratory distress syndrome (ARDS).

b) Debated – a combination of oxidative injury, cytokine-mediated damage, impaired lung protective mechanisms and pulmonary oedema. This diagnosis is the final pathway of many different aetiologies and their metabolic consequences.

c) Ventilation.
   Fluid control.
   Prevention or treatment of pulmonary hypertension.
   Exogenous surfactant.
   Pharmacological administration of T_3.
   Nitric oxide therapy.
   Oxidant scavengers.

Comments   ARDS is still poorly understood, but occurs as a result of severe pulmonary injury. The effects are probably a result of the host lung response to injury. Oxidative mechanisms are often suspected. No generally accepted treatment is available excluding general and specific supportive care. Some authorities have tried surfactant and thyroid hormones as well as nitric oxide therapy and free radical scavengers.

Answer 6.32

a) Hand and foot disease.

b) Coxsackie virus.

Comments   This infection is highly contagious. The skin manifestations include vesicular eruptions. There is no specific treatment.

Answer 6.33

a) Radioisotope bone scan.

b) Osteomyelitis of left calcaneum.

c) Intravenous antibiotics.
   Surgical drainage if necessary.

d) Monitoring of CRP levels.
   Degree of pain and activity.

Comments   The CRP is the acute phase reactant that changes most rapidly in such an infection and allows monitoring of the success of therapy. The levels rise and then fall in response to therapy faster than the ESR.

Answer 6.34

a) Polydactyly.

b) Familial, but not syndromic.
   Patau's syndrome.
   Ellis–van Creveld syndrome.
   Jeune's syndrome.
   Laurence–Moon–Biedl syndrome.
   Carpenter's syndrome.
   Orofacial digital syndrome.
   Idiopathic.

Answer 6.35

a) Bilateral pneumothoraces.

b) Reducing asynchronous ventilation: sedation; patient trigger; entraining respiratory rate; short inspiratory time; paralysis.

Comments   Pneumothoraces remain a problem in the neonatal unit. They are associated with subsequent intracranial haemorrhage. Many measures are employed to reduce the likelihood of pneumothoraces and the overall incidence is falling in most units.

6

Index

Page numbers in *italics* refer to illustrations